Updates on Hemodialysis

Edited by Ayman Karkar

Published in London, United Kingdom

Updates on Hemodialysis
http://dx.doi.org/10.5772/intechopen.105316
Edited by Ayman Karkar

Contributors
Hayfa Almutary, Saurav Singh Hamal, Pratima Khadka, Koichiro Nandate, Maiko Alejandro Alejandro Tavera Díaz, Guled Abdijalil, Nadia Kabbali, Basmat Amal Chouhani, Nidharshan S. Anandasivam, Tessa K. Novick, Ahmed Yasin, Nayer Omran, Fredrik Uhlin, Ivo Fridolin, Michael Hulko, Werner Beck, Ilona Koch, Rose Speidel, Bernd Krause, Karen Courville, Ayman Karkar

First published in London, United Kingdom, 2023 by IntechOpen
IntechOpen is the global imprint of INTECHOPEN LIMITED, registered in England and Wales, registration number: 11086078, 5 Princes Gate Court, London, SW7 2QJ, United Kingdom

British Library Cataloguing-in-Publication Data
A catalogue record for this book is available from the British Library

Additional hard and PDF copies can be obtained from orders@intechopen.com

Updates on Hemodialysis
Edited by Ayman Karkar
p. cm.
Print ISBN 978-1-80356-500-2
Online ISBN 978-1-80356-501-9
eBook (PDF) ISBN 978-1-80356-502-6

For EU product safety concerns:
IN TECH d.o.o., Prolaz Marije Krucifikse Kozulić 3, 51000 Rijeka, Croatia,
info@intechopen.com or visit our website at intechopen.com.

Meet the editor

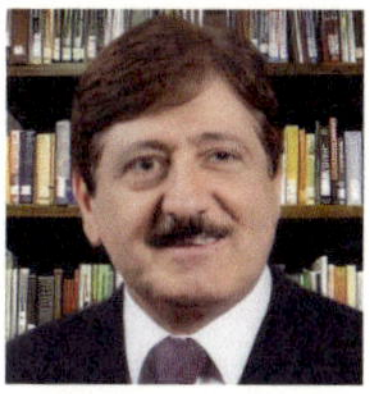

Dr. Ayman Karkar, MD, MSc, MRCP, Ph.D., FRCP, FASN, is a consultant physician and nephrologist. He is also a fellow of the Royal Colleges of Physicians (FRCP) of the United Kingdom (London), the American National Kidney Foundation, and the American Society of Nephrology. Following graduation from medical school, Dr. Karkar received his MSc in Nephology and Hypertension and Ph.D. in Renal Medicine from the Hammersmith Hospital, University of London. Dr. Karkar was a consultant physician and nephrologist at the Kanoo Kidney Centre (KKC), Dammam Medical Complex (DMC) from 2001 to 2014. He served as director of KKC and DMC in addition to supervising the renal services in the Eastern province. He was also a key advisor and chairman of numerous steering committees and provided valuable assistance, especially in setting up the dialysis outsourcing project in Saudi Arabia. Dr. Karkar is currently Baxter Head, Medical Affairs for Renal Care – Middle East and Africa. Dr. Karkar has a great interest in renal medicine and has been contributing largely to the education and training of undergraduate and postgraduate medical students and nursing staff. He has organized and participated, as a speaker or chairperson, in many congresses and symposia. Dr. Karkar is also interested in clinical research and has published around 150 papers and abstracts in peer-reviewed medical journals and 8 book chapters. He has also edited four books on renal medicine.

Contents

Preface

Hemodialysis (HD) treatment has undergone significant improvements in technology and quality performance in managing patients with kidney failure. These advancements include state-of-the-art HD machines, water treatment plants with ultrapure water, medical devices, disposables, and solutions. More recently, there have been significant improvements in the creation and maintenance of vascular access as well as the types, classifications, and monitoring of uremic toxins and their relationship with inflammation, atherosclerosis and vascular classification, and cardiovascular and all-cause mortality. Innovation in dialysis membranes/dialyzers resulted in the development of the medium cut-off membrane, which enables the removal of larger-sized uremic toxins in a safe, simple, and effective way. The HD technique that uses the medium cut-off membrane/dialyzer is known as expanded hemodialysis (HDx). HDx therapy has been shown to result in significant improvement in the quality of life of HD patients as well as reductions in hospitalization, medications, and non-fatal cardiovascular events.

Updates on Hemodialysis discusses different aspects of these innovations and can be used as a guide to improve daily practice and achieve best possible medical outcomes in HD patients. Chapters are clear and easy to read and include illustrations, figures, and tables to support the text.

I wish to thank the contributing authors for their excellent chapters. My thanks also go to IntechOpen and Publishing Process Managers Mrs. Blanka Gugic and Ms. Marina Dusevic for their assistance in collecting and editing the chapter manuscripts.

Ayman Karkar
Consultant Physician and Nephrologist,
Head Medical Affairs at Baxter International Inc.,
Renal Care – Middle East and Africa,
Dubai, United Arab Emirates

Chapter 1

Introductory Chapter: Updates on Hemodialysis

Ayman Karkar

1. Introduction

Despite the significant improvements in hemodialysis (HD) techniques over the past 40 years, patients on this therapy still suffer from the burden of HD-associated symptoms, vascular access-related issues, acute and chronic complications, poor quality of life, and the mortality rate remains unacceptably elevated [1, 2]. The European Renal Association (ERA) and the United States Renal Data System (USRDS) showed that the 5-year survival rate for patients on HD is close to only 50%, which is worse than patients with breast cancer, prostate cancer and almost like or worse than colon cancer [3–6].

The retention of large-size uremic toxins (e.g., proinflammatory cytokines, alpha 1-microglobulin, YKL-40, and kappa and lambda free light chains) has been associated with inflammation, atherosclerosis and vascular calcification, cardiovascular disease, and increased risk of mortality [7]. These uremic toxins have also been associated with poor quality of life, such as late recovery time post-HD session, impaired physical function, moderate-to-severe pruritus, and restless legs syndrome [8]. These drawbacks of HD treatment demonstrate the unmet needs in the current or conventional HD modalities.

2. Uremic toxins and hemodialysis techniques

The new medium cut-off membrane/dialyzer, with its larger pore size, lower wall thickness, and smaller inner diameter of hollow fibers, has significantly improved the clearance of the large-size uremic toxins in safe, simple, and effective technique, especially when compared to conventional hemodialysis techniques [9]. For example, the low-flux HD can remove small soluble solutes less than 500 Dalton (Da), such as urea and creatinine, whereas high-flux HD is capable of efficiently removing molecules less than 15,000 Da. Diffusion is the major contributor to the clearance of small-size molecules, but convection, as in online hemodiafiltration (HDF), is required for the efficient removal of large-size molecules, especially those above 25,000 Da [7]. Randomized controlled trials have shown the effectiveness of online HDF not only in its ability to remove large-size uremic toxins but to improve the quality of life [10] and to significantly reduce the cardiovascular and all-cause mortality, especially if the used prescribed convection volume equals to or exceeds 23 liters/1.73 m^2/session [11]. However, successful implementation of online HDF is demanding. For example, it requires a special HD machine that has the ability to mix solutions online, a powerful high-flux dialyzer, functional vascular access with a blood flow rate of 350–400 ml/

IntechOpen

minute (difficult with central venous catheters or not properly functioning arteriovenous fistula or graft), consumption of large volume of water (almost double what is needed for conventional HD), ultrapure water (free from bacteria and endotoxin), frequent monitoring of water quality, training of medical and nursing staff (especially when the turnover is frequent) and achievement of the prescribed convective volume [12].

The actual value of the medium cut-off membrane/dialyzer is its ability to perform diffusion and convection with fluid replacement (internal filtration) internally simulating, and probably more effective than, online HDF, without the need for external replacement fluids [13], using a basic HD machine with a blood flow rate of 250–300 ml/minute [14], and standard water quality (ISO11663 or ANSI/AAMI RD62) [15–21] for conventional HD over the 4-hours dialysis session. This modality of HD is referred to as HDx or expanded hemodialysis [9]. HDx therapy has been shown to remove effectively larger-size uremic toxins [22], improvement of quality of life [23–26], reduction in HD-related medications (e.g., erythropoietin and iron) [27, 28], and a significant decrease in hospitalization rate [29, 30] and nonfatal cardiovascular disease [18].

3. Complications of hemodialysis

The technique of hemodialysis, especially with the recent developments in the technology of HD machines, is still associated with several acute and chronic complications, such as intradialytic hypotension, hypertension, fluid retention, risk of bleeding (among other hematological complications), muscle cramps, arrhythmias, and sudden cardiac death. "*Updates on Hemodialysis*" reviews and updates the reader on these complications, and some iatrogenic errors such as hypernatremia, iron overload, pseudoaneurysm, and air embolism. Hemodialysis patients also suffer from and are affected by different psychological stresses upon starting dialysis and during the course of treatment, which affect different lifestyle changes. The "*Updates on Hemodialysis*" describes the most common psychosocial issues among patients on hemodialysis treatment.

4. Vascular access

There are three types of vascular access. These are arteriovenous fistula, arteriovenous graft, and central venous catheters. Each of these has its uses and advantages and disadvantages. Vascular access is the lifeline for patients in need of hemodialysis. "*Updates on Hemodialysis*" reviews the basics of perioperative anesthetic management, including the choice of anesthesia method, pre-anesthesia preparation, intraoperative and postoperative management, and the effect of choice of anesthesia on the outcomes. In addition, "*Updates on Hemodialysis*" updates the reader on recent innovations in central venous catheter's tip and coating designs, newer arteriovenous fistula access techniques, including a percutaneous endovascular method, innovations in arteriovenous graft, including drug-eluting devices that may reduce neointimal hyperplasia and bioengineered blood vessels, and arteriovenous graft/central venous catheter device, which enables bypassing vessel stenoses.

The "*Updates on Hemodialysis*" book aims at reviewing and updating the reader on understanding type, source, classification of uremic toxins, and ways of their monitoring, HD-related complications, hypertension in HD, errors in HD practices, and psychological status of HD patients, management and innovation of vascular access techniques, resistance to erythropoietin and its prescription, and extracorporeal management of liver failure. "*Updates on Hemodialysis*" book has also focused on the recent innovation in dialysis membranes/dialyzers, particularly the medium cut-off membrane and its ability to remove the larger-size uremic toxins more efficiently in a HD modality known as expanded hemodialysis (HDx).

Author details

Ayman Karkar
Medical Affairs - Renal Care, Dubai, United Arab Emirates

*Address all correspondence to: han94dan97@gmail.com

References

[1] Zhang JC, El-Majzoub S, Li M, Ahmed T, Wu J, Lipman ML, et al. Could symptom burden predict subsequent healthcare use in patients with end stage kidney disease on hemodialysis care? A prospective, preliminary study. Renal Failure. 2020;**42**(1):294-301. DOI: 10.1080/0886022X.2020.1744449

[2] Ashuntantang G, Osafo C, Olowu WA, Arogundade F, Niang A, Porter J, et al. Outcomes in adults and children with end-stage kidney disease requiring dialysis in sub-Saharan Africa: A systematic review. The Lancet Global Health. 2017;**5**(4):e408-e417. DOI: 10.1016/S2214-109X(17)30057-8

[3] Collins AJ, Foley RN, Herzog C, Chavers B, Gilbertson D, Ishani A, et al. United States renal data system 2008 annual data report. American Journal of Kidney Diseases. 2009;**53**(1 Suppl):S1-S374. DOI: 10.1053/j.ajkd.2008.10.005

[4] ERA-EDTA Registry: ERA-EDTA Registry Annual Report 2012. EUROCARE-5 database. Available from: http://www.eurocare.it/Eurocare5/tabid/64/Default.aspx [Accessed: February 18, 2023]

[5] United States Renal Data System. 2018 USRDS Annual Data Report: End-Stage Renal Disease in the United States. Bethesda, MD: National Institutes of Health, National Institute of Diabetes and Digestive and Kidney Diseases; 2018

[6] Noone AM, Cronin KA, Altekruse SF, Howlader N, Lewis DR, Petkov VI, et al. SEER Cancer Statistics Review, 1975-2015, National Cancer Institute, Bethesda, MD. Based on November 2017 SEER data submission, posted to the SEER website April 2018;**3**. Available from: http://seer.cancer.gov/csr/1975_2015/

[7] Rosner MH, Reis T, Husain-Syed F, Vanholder R, Hutchison C, Stenvinkel P, et al. Classification of uremic toxins and their role in kidney failure. Clinical Journal of the American Society of Nephrology. 2021;**16**:1918-1928. DOI: 10.2215/CJN.02660221

[8] Sapa H, Gutierrez OM, Shlipak MG, Katz R, Ix JH, Sarnak MJ, et al. Association of uremic solutes with cardiovascular death in diabetic kidney disease. American Journal of Kidney Diseases. **80**(4):502-512. DOI: 10.1053/j.ajkd.2022.02.016

[9] Ronco C. The rise of expanded hemodialysis. Blood Purification. 2017;**44**(2):I-VIII. DOI: 10.1159/000476012

[10] Karkar A, Abdelrahman M, Locatelli F. A randomized trial on health-related patients satisfaction level with high-efficiency online hemodiafiltration versus high-flux hemodialysis. Blood Purification. 2015;**40**:84-91. DOI: 10.1159/000381255

[11] Peters SAE, Bots ML, Canaud B, Davenport A, Grooteman MPC, Kircelli F, et al. Haemodiafiltration and mortality in end-stage kidney disease patients: A pooled individual participant data analysis from four randomized controlled trials. Nephrology Dialysis Transplantation. 2016;**31**:978-984. DOI: 10.1093/ndt/gfv349

[12] Karkar A. Chapter: Introduction to hemodiafiltration. In: Karkar A, editor. Advances in Hemodiafiltration. London, UK: INTECH Hemodiafiltration Book; 2016. ISBN 978-953-51-2562-4

[13] Lorenzin A, Golino G, de Cal M, Pajarin G, Savastano S, Lupi A, et al. Flow dynamic analysis by contrast-enhanced imaging techniques of

medium cutoff membrane hemodialyzer. Blood Purification. 2022;**51**:138-146. DOI: 10.1159/000516411

[14] Kim TH, Kim SH, Kim TY, Park HY, Jung KS, Lee MH, et al. Removal of large middle molecules via haemodialysis with medium cut-off membranes at lower blood flow rates: An observational prospective study. BMC Nephrology. 2020;**21**:2. DOI: 10.1186/s12882-019-1669-3

[15] Schepers E, Glorieux G, Eloot S, Hulko M, Boschetti-de-Fierro A, Beck W, et al. Assessment of the association between increasing membrane pore size and endotoxin permeability using a novel experimental dialysis simulation set-up. BMC Nephrology. 2018;**19**(1):1. DOI: 10.1186/s12882-017-0808-y

[16] Hulko M, Dietrich V, Koch I, Gekeler A, Gebert M, Beck W, et al. Pyrogen retention: Comparison of the novel medium cut-off (MCO) membrane with other dialyser membranes. Scientific Reports. 2019;**9**(1):6791. DOI: 10.1038/s41598-019-43161-2

[17] Weiner DE, Falzon L, Skoufos L, Bernardo A, Beck W, Xiao M, et al. Efficacy and safety of expanded hemodialysis with the theranova 400 dialyzer: A randomized controlled trial. Clinical Journal of the American Society of Nephrology. 2020;**15**(9):1310-1319. DOI: 10.2215/CJN.01210120

[18] Molano AP, Hutchison CA, Sanchez R, Rivera AS, Buitrago G, Dazzarola MP, et al. Medium cutoff versus high-flux hemodialysis membranes and clinical outcomes: A cohort study using inverse probability treatment weighting. Kidney Medicine. 2022;**4**(4):100431. DOI: 10.1016/j.xkme.2022.100431

[19] European Best Practice Guidelines for Hemodialysis. Section IV. Dialysis fluid purity. Nephrology, Dialysis, Transplantation. 2002;**17**:45-62

[20] AAMI Renal Disease and Detoxification Committee. Dialysate for Hemodialysis. Arlington, VA: AAMI; 2004. pp. 24-27

[21] American National Standard Institute, American Association for medical Instrumentation, International Standard Organization 13959. 2014: Water for Hemodialysis and Related Therapies

[22] Kirsch AH, Lyko R, Nilsson LR, Beck W, Amdahl M, Lechner P, et al. Performance of hemodialysis with novel medium cut-off dialyzers. Nephrology Dialysis Transplantation. 2017;**32**:165-172. DOI: 10.1093/ndt/gfw310

[23] Alarcon JC, Bunch A, Ardila F, Zuñiga E, Vesga JI, Rivera A, et al. Impact of medium cut-off dialyzers on patient-reported outcomes: COREXH registry. Blood Purification. 2021;**50**:110-118. DOI: 10.1159/000508803

[24] Bolton S, Gair R, Nilsson LG, Matthews M, Stewart L, McCullagh N. Clinical assessment of dialysis recovery time and symptom burden: Impact of switching hemodialysis therapy mode. Patient Related Outcome Measures (Dovepress). 2021;**12**:315-321. DOI: 10.2147/PROM.S325016

[25] Penny JD, Jarosz P, Salerno FR, Lemoine S, McIntyre CW. Impact of expanded hemodialysis using medium cut-off dialyzer on quality of life: Application of dynamic patient-reported outcome measurement tool. Kidney Medicine. 2021;**3**(6):992-1002. DOI: 10.1016/j.xkme.2021.05.010

[26] Lim JH, Park Y, Yook JM, Choi SY, Hee-HY, Choi JY, et al. Randomized controlled trial of medium cut-off versus high-flux dialyzers on quality

of life outcomes in maintenance hemodialysis patients. Scientific Reports. 2020;**10**:7780. DOI: 10.1038/s41598-020-64622-z

[27] Lim JH, Jeon Y, Yook JM, Choi SY, Jung HY, Choi JY, et al. Medium cut-off dialyzer improves erythropoiesis stimulating agent resistance in a hepcidin-independent manner in maintenance hemodialysis patients: Results from a randomized controlled trial. Scientific Reports. 2020;**10**:16062. DOI: 10.1038/s41598-020-73124-x

[28] Hadad-Arrascue F, Nilsson LG, Rivera AS, Bernardo AA, Romero JBC. Expanded hemodialysis as effective alternative to on-line hemodiafiltration: A randomized mid-term clinical trial. Therapeutic Apheresis and Dialysis. 2021:1-8. DOI: 10.1111/1744-9987.13700

[29] Blackowicz MJ, Falzon L, Beck W, Tran H, Weiner DE. Economic evaluation of expanded hemodialysis with the Theranova 400 dialyzer: A post hoc evaluation of a randomized clinical trial in the United States. Hemodialysis International. 2022:1-7. DOI: 10.1111/hdi.13015

[30] Sanabria RM, Hutchison CA, Vesga JI, Ariza JG, Sanchez R, Suarez AM. Expanded hemodialysis and its effects on hospitalizations and medication usage: A cohort study. Nephron. 2021;**145**:179-187. DOI: 10.1159/000513328

Chapter 2

Uremic Toxins: The Role of the Gut and the Kidneys

Karen Courville

Abstract

Uremic toxins are a diverse group of substances that contribute significantly to the high cardiovascular disease burden in chronic kidney disease (CKD). When glomerular filtration begins to decrease, a disorder in the intestinal microflora known as dysbiosis occurs; this produces alterations in metabolic activities and decreased excretion of waste products. These substances have been identified and classified, accordingly to molecular weight and clearance. Biological and clinical effects have also been identified. These substances have different effects depending on the tissue or cell where they accumulate. The recommendations for a low-protein diet in pre-dialysis patients and the use of probiotics, prebiotics, and synbiotics added to the removal techniques in hemodialysis can help reduce the inflammatory effects and those associated with mortality.

Keywords: uremic toxins, chronic kidney disease, dysbiosis, hemodialysis, cardiovascular mortality

1. Introduction

Uremic toxins are substances produced by protein metabolism. In persons with chronic kidney disease (CKD), these substances can accumulate and contribute to the diversity of symptoms produced by end-stage kidney disease.

In the gut, protein metabolism by bacteria produces ammonia, in the presence of urease enzymes. Diet has an important role, as animal protein generates more uremic toxins than vegetable proteins. Also, microbial fermentation of some amino acids and gut microbes can generate uremic toxins.

Patients with advanced chronic kidney disease in pre-dialysis and patients in renal replacement therapy need an adequate balance of protein in the diet, since dialysis can remove some uremic toxins, but not all and studies suggest that these toxins can contribute to cardiovascular risk and mortality.

2. Dysbiosis in chronic kidney disease

Uremic toxins are substances produced by protein metabolism. This substance accumulates in patients with chronic kidney disease (CKD) and produce deterioration of physiologic and biochemical functions that contribute to gastrointestinal symptoms, malnutrition, and progression of end-stage kidney disease [1].

Under normal circumstances, native bacteria are acquired at birth and during the first year of life, and some other transit bacteria are acquired during our daily food and fluid intake. Acids and bile from gastric and pancreatic enzymes secretion prevent most bacteria to grow in the first part of the gastrointestinal tract; but from past the duodenum until the distal colon, there is a population of some 100 billions bacteria that live in symbiosis with the human host [2], and that studies have shown that have roles in metabolic and nutritional function; protection from invasive infectious agents; proliferation and differentiation of intestinal epithelia; and modulation of immune system [3].

Approximately, 10 g of protein reaches the colon daily, where it is broken down by gut bacteria to metabolites such as ammonium, amines, thiols, phenols, and indoles. These products are normally eliminated by the feces, and a part are absorbed and eliminated by the kidney [4].

With progression of CKD, disorders of the intestinal microflora occur (dysbiosis), and there is an alteration in the quantity and quality of its composition and metabolic activities [5]. Rising urea levels and the spread of urease bacteria increase ammonium production in the intestinal lumen and induce changes in intestinal pH, altering the permeability of the intestinal mucosa, by affecting the enterocytes in the tight junction, producing an infiltration of mononuclear leukocytes in the lamina propria that is associated with an increased thickening of the colonic wall [6].

In addition to the decrease in the clearance of waste products, CKD patients use multiple medications, have a decrease in dietary fiber consumption, and need oral iron and frequent use of antibiotics that also produce alterations in intestinal transit [7]. Patients in hemodialysis have episodes of hypervolemia alternated with ultrafiltration and, sometimes, hypotension that can cause episodes of transient intestinal ischemia and also increase the permeability of the intestinal barrier and, with this, favor the passage of endotoxins [6].

There are more than 100 substances that have been identified as uremic toxins, and studies continue to suggest more each day. There are some characteristics that these substances must meet to be considered as uremic toxins: identification and measurement should be possible and levels should be elevated in CKD patients and when decreased, symptoms should improve [8–10].

There are differences in their physicochemical characteristics, as size, weight and clearance, and site of origin, that have allowed them to be classified into small water-soluble, small middle, medium-middle size, large-middle molecules, and protein-bound compounds. Some of these compounds are derived from endogenous metabolism and are water-soluble, but some are gut derived from dysbiosis and can be water-soluble or protein-bound (**Table 1**) [11, 12].

2.1 Small molecules (water-soluble and protein-bound)

The water-soluble small molecules have the characteristic that they can be easily removed with any type of dialysis (low-flux hemodialysis). Among these, we have creatine, creatinine, urea, and uric acid. The protein-bound small molecules, such as indoxyl sulfate, P-cresyl sulfate, and homocysteine, are difficult to remove by available dialysis techniques and are known to have toxic activity. Studies have confirmed

Small molecules Water soluble Protein bound[**] (< 0.5 kDa) (Gut derived) Low flux HD[*] MCO HDx	**Small-middle Molecules (0.5–15 kDa) High flux HD[*]**	**Medium-middle Molecule Compounds (>15–25 kDa) High flux HDF[*]**	**Large-middle molecules (25–58 kDa) MCO HDx[*]**	**Large molecules >58 HCO HD[*]**
Carbamylated compounds	B2-microglobuline	IL-1β, IL-6, IL-10 IL-18	AOPP	Modified albumin
ADMA	IL-8	myoglobin	FGF-23	
urea		Kappa-FLC	Lambda-FLC	
Uric acid		prolactin	TNFR1	
TMAO		TNF-α	AGEs	
SDMA		Complement factor D	CX3CL1	
Indoxyl sulfate[**]		FGF-2	CXCL12	
P-cresyl sulfate[**]			IL-2	
Homocysteine[**]			YKL-40	

ADMA: asymmetric dimethylarginine; TMAO: trimethylamine-N-oxide, SDMA: symmetric dimethylarginine; FLC: free light chain; TNF: tumor necrosis factor; FGF: Fibroblast growth factor; AOPP: Advanced oxidative protein products; IL: Interleukin; AGEs: Advanced glycation end products; CX: chemokine; and YKL: chitinase like protein.
[*]All dialyzer types can remove small water soluble compounds, but for each molecular weight group, there is a dialysis modality with a higher capacity to remove each group of compounds: HD: hemodialysis; HDF: hemodiafiltration; MCO medium cutoff; HDx: expanded hemodialysis; HCO: high cutoff.
[**]Molecules removed by MCO HDx.
Adapted from: Rosner et al. [12].

Table 1.
Classification of uremic toxins.

that these molecules get better removal with a medium cutoff (MCO) membrane and expanded hemodialysis (HDx) [13, 14].

There are different indoles substances, produced by degradation of tryptophan by intestinal bacteria and subsequently sulfated in the liver. Indoxyl sulfate has been found to be the most abundant in uremic patients [15]. Studies have demonstrated a relation with renal fibrosis and progression of end-stage renal disease and an association with endothelial damage, as this substance can inhibit endothelial repair functions and free radical production [16].

P-cresol is a phenol produced by the metabolism of phenylalanine and tyrosine and then conjugated in the intestinal wall to p-cresyl sulfate and to p-cresyl glucuronide in the liver, being p-cresyl sulfate the main metabolite circulating in the cresol group [17].

2.2 Small middle molecules

These substances have a higher molecular weight. β2-microglobuline, PTH, and IL-8 can be removed by using high-flux hemodialysis (HD-high flux). The accumulation of β2-microglobuline in osteoarticular or viscera is known as dialysis-associated amyloidosis, and deposits contributes to destructive lesions of bones and joints and vascular damage [18].

2.3 Medium middle molecules

These molecules can be removed from plasma by using convective (hemofiltration or hemodiafiltration) or large-pore membrane dialysis techniques, such as peritoneal dialysis and high-flux hemodialysis. Some of these are myoglobin, prolactin, interleukins (IL-1B, IL-6, IL-10, and IL-18), and Kappa-free light chain, and they contribute to maintaining a state of chronic inflammation [19].

2.4 Large middle molecules

These group of molecules are composed by cytokines, growth factors, and signaling proteins; but since they are retained in uremia and clearance for these molecules is difficult with low-flux hemodialysis techniques, the accumulation of these substances is associated with endothelial dysfunction and cardiovascular disease [20].

2.5 Large molecules

In this group, we find that albumin, but in the presence of uremia, suffers an irreversible nonenzymatic post-translational modification, called carbamylation, that is associated with pro-atherogenic, endothelial dysfunction, monocyte adhesion, and cardiovascular mortality [21].

3. Biological and clinical effects of uremic toxins

The fermentation of non-digestible carbohydrates takes places mainly in the cecum and right colon. For bacteria, this is an important source of energy for proliferation and energy recovery from the diet that favors the absorption of ions (Ca, Ng, and Fe) in the cecum. The enteric flora also helps in the production of vitamins (K, B12, biotin, folic, and pantothenic acid) and the synthesis of amino acids from ammonia or urea [22]. Anaerobic metabolism of peptides and proteins that occur in distal segments of the colon generates ammonia, amines, phenols, thiols, and indoles [23].

There are some factors that favor bacterial translocation: bacterial proliferation in small intestine, increased permeability of the mucosal barrier, and deficiencies in immune response. CKD patients share those factors that can contribute to accumulation of uremic toxins [24].

Uremic toxins have different effects at tissue and cellular levels. At the endothelial level, there is an alteration in the balance of nitric oxide production, and there is an increase in the production of free oxygen radicals, inflammation, proliferation, and expression of tissue factor and ICAM-1 and MCP-1 [25]. In the smooth vascular fiber, there is production of free radicals and proliferation and an increase in the expression of osteoblastic proteins. Increased calcification, aortic stiffness, atherosclerosis, and increased leukocyte adhesion to the wall have been seen in the blood vessels [26].

In cardiac myocytes, the presence of these toxins causes alterations in cellular structure and function and has been associated with cardiac hypertrophy and fibrosis [27]. In bone, there are alterations in the differentiation and function of osteoclasts, and in osteoblasts, there is a decrease in the expression of the PTH receptor, with a decrease in cell viability and proliferation [28]; in adipocytes, deposits of uremic toxins have been associated with insulin resistance [29].

Uremic toxins have been associated with progression of end-stage kidney disease, cardiovascular complications, and alterations of mineral-bone metabolism, anemia, and insulin resistance. The deposits in the glomeruli, tubules, and interstitium produce monocyte infiltration, glomerulosclerosis, and tubulointerstitial fibrosis [30, 31]. There is interference in the production of erythropoietin, added to a decrease in the life of erythrocytes, which has been related to renal patient anemia [32, 33].

4. Treatment recommendations

It has been seen in general terms that the inhibition of the production of uremic toxins derived from the production of intestinal bacteria may have a potential use. There are certain bacteria that assist the small intestine; however, if its population is depleted or otherwise overstimulated and grows, then an increase in population may also cause a problem. There are some potential therapeutic effects on using decreasing the amount of protein in the diet and the use of some substances (**Table 2**) [34].

4.1 Low-protein diets

Low-protein diets could be helpful, since by decreasing the intake of amino acids, the production of uremic substances can be reduced. Diets with animal protein (meat) increase the production of nitrogenous waste products, increase the risk of constipation, and worsen uremia. Strategies to reduce the amount of animal protein and increase the intake of vegetable protein may have an impact on decreasing glomerular hyperfiltration [35].

It has been evaluated that low-protein diets can slow the progression of chronic kidney disease. However, patients do not reach the goal stipulated in the recommendations of low-protein diets of 0.6–0.8 g/kg/day. One strategy would be to supplement diets with essential amino acids or ketoanalogs [36]. It is important that diets for patients must be modulated, since a very strict diet could lead the patient to a state of malnutrition [37].

4.2 Probiotics

Probiotics are a group of living species of known bacteria (*Lactobacillus acidophilus*, *bifidobacterium longum*, and *streptococci*) that administered orally and have shown to decrease some levels of potentially toxic substances such as homocysteine, indoxyl sulfate, cytokines (TNF-α, IL-5, IL-6), and pro-inflammatory endotoxins in patients with chronic kidney disease [38–40].

Low protein diet	Probiotics	Prebiotics	Synbiotics
Reduce production of nitrogenous waste products	Decrease production of toxic products and endotoxins	Modification of gut environment	Improving survival of intestinal bacteria
Decrease in production of toxic waste products and inflammatory substances			

Table 2.
Suggested treatment strategies.

4.3 Prebiotics

Prebiotics are a non-digestible food ingredient that promotes the growth of beneficial microorganisms in the intestines. The majority of them are a subset of carbohydrate groups and oligosaccharide carbohydrates (OSCs), like fructo-oligosaccharides and galacto-oligosaccharides. By providing energy sources for the gut microbiota, prebiotics can modulate the composition and function of these microorganisms and can modify the gut environment [41]. The fermentation products of prebiotics are mostly acidic, thus lowering the intestinal pH. This can contribute to a change in the composition and population of the intestinal microbiota, and in some cases, the fermentation of a prebiotic complex is a substrate for another microorganism [42]. Prebiotics are found in fruits, vegetables, and whole grains like apples, artichokes, asparagus, bananas, barley, wheat, oat, onions, and green vegetables but are also added to some foods. The use of prebiotics decreases the production of indoles and p-cresyl sulfate due to the production of short-chain fatty acids (SCFAs), which provides energy to the intestine, and allows the amino acids that reach the colon to be incorporated into the bacteria and therefore excreted, instead of being used to generate uremic solutes [43].

4.4 Synbiotics

Synbiotics are substances that contain a mixture of probiotics and prebiotics, with the intention of improving the activity and survival of bacteria in the intestine. Several studies in patients with stage 3 to 5 chronic kidney disease have evaluated some synbiotic-type products, managing to find a decrease in the values of uremic toxins in the blood. Reports of some laxatives agents [44] and oral activated charcoal adsorbent AST-120 [45] have suggested to reduce concentrations of some uremic toxins, but the effect wanes after stopping its use. Some studies in animals with chronic kidney disease have evaluated the use of sodium-glucose cotransporter (SGLT) 2 inhibitor Canagliflozin. This drug also has an inhibitory effect on SGLT 1, which has a gastrointestinal effect by promoting intestinal fermentation of carbohydrates and reducing plasma levels of p-cresyl and indoles [46, 47].

5. Conclusions

There is abundant evidence in the literature that the retention of uremic toxins contributes to generalized inflammatory damage in patients with chronic kidney disease [48]. The general recommendation of a balanced diet, with a low amount of protein and an adequate amount of fiber, depending on the renal stage, is important. Bacterial overgrowth produces retention of uremic toxins that cause intestinal dysbiosis. All the strategies that can be used to preserve residual renal function or reduce cellular inflammation are important to complete a multidisciplinary approach for the management of CKD that increasingly affects more and more patients worldwide.

Acknowledgment

Dr. Courville is a member of the Sistema Nacional de Investigadores SNI which is supported by Panama's Secretaría Nacional de Cienia y Tecnología SENACYT.

DOI: http://dx.doi.org/10.5772/intechopen.109845

Author details

Karen Courville
Section of Nephrology, Department of Medicine, Hospital Dr. Gustavo Nelson Collado, Chitré, Herrera, Panama

*Address all correspondence to: kavac7@gmail.com

References

[1] Glassock RJ. Uremic toxins: What are they? An integrated overview of pathobiology and classification. Journal of Renal Nutrition. 2008;**18**(1):2-6. DOI: 10.1053/j.jrn.2007.10.003

[2] Tannock GW. What immunologists should know about bacterial communities of the human bowel. Seminars in Immunology. 2007;**19**(2):94-105. DOI: 10.1016/j.smim.2006.09.001. Epub 2006 Oct 10

[3] Guarner F, Malagelada JR. Gut flora in health and disease. Lancet. 2003;**361**(9356):512-519. DOI: 10.1016/S0140-6736(03)12489-0

[4] Evenepoel P, Meijers BK, Bammens BR, Verbeke K. Uremic toxins originating from colonic microbial metabolism. Kidney International. Supplement. 2009;**114**:S12-S19. DOI: 10.1038/ki.2009.402

[5] Meijers B, Evenepoel P, Anders HJ. Intestinal microbiome and fitness in kidney disease. Nature Reviews. Nephrology. 2019;**15**:531-545

[6] Vaziri ND. CKD impairs barrier function and alters microbial flora of the intestine: A major link to inflammation and uremic toxicity. Current Opinion in Nephrology and Hypertension. 2012;**21**(6):587-592. DOI: 10.1097/MNH.0b013e328358c8d5

[7] Bloor SR, Schutte R, Hobson AR. Oral Iron Supplementation—Gastrointestinal Side Effects and the Impact on the Gut Microbiota. Microbiology Research. 2021;**12**(2):491-502

[8] Vanholder R, Van Laecke S, Glorieux G. What is new in uremic toxicity? Pediatric Nephrology. 2008;**23**(8):1211-1221. DOI: 10.1007/s00467-008-0762-9. Epub 2008 Mar 7

[9] Vanholder R, De Smet R, Glorieux G, Argiles A, Baurmeister U, Brunet P, et al. European uremic toxin work group (EUTox) review on uremic toxins: Classification, concentration, and interindividual variability. Kidney International. 2003;**63**(5):1934-1943

[10] Vanholder R, Baurmeister U, Brunet P, Cohen G, Glorieux G, Jankowski J. European uremic toxin work group: A bench to bedside view of uremic toxins. Journal of the American Society of Nephrology. 2008;**19**:863-870

[11] Meert N, Schepers E, Glorieux G, Van Landschoot M, Goeman HL, Waterloss M-A, et al. Novel method for simultaneous determination of p-cresylsulphate and p-cresylglucoronide: Clinical data and pathophysiological implications. Nephrology, Dialysis, Transplantation. 2012;**27**:2388-2396

[12] Rosner M, Reis T, Husain-Syed F, Vanholder R, Hutchinson C, Stenvinkel P, et al. Classification of uremic toxins and their role in kidney failure. Clinical Journal of the American Society of Nephrology. 2021;**16**:1918-1928

[13] Ronco C, La Manna G. Expanded hemodialysis: A new therapy for a new class of membranas. Contributions to Nephrology. 2017;**190**:124-133

[14] Zhang Z, Yang T, Li Y, Li J, Yang Q, Wang L, et al. Effects of expanded hemodialysis with medium cut-off membranes on maintenance hemodialysis patients: A review. Membranes. 2022;**12**(3):253

[15] Dou L, Bertrand E, Cerini C, Faure V, Sampol J, Vanholder R, et al. The uremic

solutes p-cresol and indoxyl sulfate inhibit endothelial proliferation and wound repair. Kidney International. 2004;**65**(2):442-451

[16] Dou L, Jourde-Chiche N, Faure V, Cerini C, Berland Y, Dignat-George F, et al. The uremic solute indoxyl sulfate induces oxidative stress in endothelial cells. Journal of Thrombosis and Haemostasis. 2007;**5**(6):1302-1308

[17] Martinez AW, Recht NS, Hostetter TH, Meyer TW. Removal of P-cresol sulfate by hemodialysis. Journal of the American Society of Nephrology. 2005;**16**(11):3430-3436. DOI: 10.1681/ASN.2005030310

[18] Scarpioni R, Ricardi M, Albertazzi V, De Amicis S, Rastelli F, Zerbini L. Dialysis-related amyloidosis: Challenges and solutions. International Journal of Nephrology and Renovascular Disease. 2016;**9**:319-328

[19] Nlandu Y, Padden M, Seidowsky A, Hamaz S, Vilaine É, Cheddani L, et al. Toxines urémiques de moyen poids moléculaire : un véritable regain d'intérêt [Middle-molecule uremic toxins: A renewed interest]. Néphrologie & Thérapeutique. 2019;**15**(2):82-90

[20] Wolley MJ, Hutchison CA. Large uremic toxins: An unsolved problem in end-stage kidney disease. Nephrology, Dialysis, Transplantation. 2018;**33**(suppl_3):iii6-iii11

[21] Gorisse L, Jaisson S, Piétrement C, Gillery P. Carbamylated proteins in renal disease: Aggravating factors or just biomarkers? International Journal of Molecular Sciences. 2022;**23**(1):574

[22] Hooper LV, Midtvedt T, Gordon JI. How host-microbial interactions shape the nutrient environment of the mammalian intestine. Annual Review of Nutrition. 2002;**22**:283-307

[23] Macfarlane GT, Macfarlane S. Bacteria, colonic fermentation, and gastrointestinal health. Journal of AOAC International. 2012;**95**(1):50-60. DOI: 10.5740/jaoacint.sge_macfarlane

[24] Guarner F. Papel de la flora intestinal en la salud y en la enfermedad. Nutrición Hospitalaria. 2007;**22**(Suppl. 2):14-19

[25] Felipe I, Castellaro BC. La Vasculatura Sistémica En La Enfermedad Renal Crónica. Primera Parte. Rev. nefrol. dial. traspl. 2019;**39**(4):279-290. Available from: http://www.scielo.org.ar/scielo.php?script=sci_arttext&pid=S2346-85482019000400279&lng=es

[26] Stubbs JR, House JA, Ocque AJ, Zhang S, Johnson C, Kimber C, et al. Serum trimethylamine-N-oxide is elevated in CKD and correlates with coronary atherosclerosis burden. Journal of the American Society of Nephrology. 2016;**27**(1):305-313. DOI: 10.1681/ASN.2014111063

[27] Biagi E, Nylund L, Candela M, Ostan R, Bucci L, Pini E, et al. Through ageing, and beyond: Gut microbiota and inflammatory status in seniors and centenarians. PLoS One. 2010;**5**(5):e10667. DOI: 10.1371/journal.pone.0010667

[28] Nii-Kono T, Iwasaki Y, Uchida M, Fujieda A, Hosokawa A, Motojima M, et al. Indoxyl sulfate induces skeletal resistance to parathyroid hormone in cultured osteoblastic cells. Kidney International. 2007;**71**(8):738-743. DOI: 10.1038/sj.ki.5002097

[29] Soulage CO, Koppe L, Fouque D. Protein-bound uremic toxins...new targets to prevent insulin resistance and dysmetabolism in patients with chronic kidney disease. Journal of Renal Nutrition. 2013;**23**(6):464-466. DOI: 10.1053/j.jrn.2013.06.003

[30] Motojima M, Hosokawa A, Yamato H, Muraki T, Yoshioka T. Uremic toxins of organic anions up-regulate PAI-1 expression by induction of NF-kappaB and free radical in proximal tubular cells. Kidney International. 2003;**63**(5):1671-1680. DOI: 10.1046/j. 1523-1755.2003.00906.x

[31] Mutsaers HA, Stribos EG, Glorieux G, Vanholder R, Olinga P. Chronic kidney disease and fibrosis: The role of uremic retention solutes. Frontiers in Medicine (Lausanne). 2015;**2**:60. DOI: 10.3389/fmed.2015.00060

[32] Nangaku M, Mimura I, Yamaguchi J, Higashijima Y, Wada T, Tanaka T. Role of uremic toxins in erythropoiesis-stimulating agent resistance in chronic kidney disease and dialysis patients. Journal of Renal Nutrition. 2015;**25**(2):160-163. DOI: 10.1053/j. jrn.2014.10.011

[33] Ahmed MS, Abed M, Voelkl J, Lang F. Triggering of suicidal erythrocyte death by uremic toxin indoxyl sulfate. BMC Nephrology. 2013;**14**:244. DOI: 10.1186/ 1471-2369-14-244

[34] Kalantar-Zadeh K, Joshi S, Schlueter R, Cooke J, Brown-Tortorici A, Donnelly M, et al. Plant-dominant low-protein diet for conservative management of chronic kidney disease. Nutrients. 2020;**12**(7):1931. DOI: 10.3390/nu12071931

[35] Ko GJ, Obi Y, Tortorici AR, Kalantar-Zadeh K. Dietary protein intake and chronic kidney disease. Current Opinion in Clinical Nutrition and Metabolic Care. 2017;**20**(1):77-85. DOI: 10.1097/MCO.0000000000000342

[36] Lim YJ, Sidor NA, Tonial NC, Che A, Urquhart BL. Uremic toxins in the progression of chronic kidney disease and cardiovascular disease: Mechanisms and therapeutic targets. Toxins (Basel). 2021;**13**(2):142. DOI: 10.3390/ toxins13020142

[37] Rastall RA, Gibson GR, Gill HS, Guarner F, Klaenhammer TR, Pot B, et al. Modulation of the microbial ecology of the human colon by probiotics, prebiotics and synbiotics to enhance human health: An overview of enabling science and potential applications. FEMS Microbiology Ecology. 2005;**52**:145-152

[38] Van Baarlen P, Troost FJ, Van Hemert S, van der Meer C, de Vos WM, de Groot PJ, et al. Differential NF-κB pathways induction by *lactobacillus plantarum* in the duodenum of healthy humans correlating with immune tolerance. Proceedings of the National Academy of Sciences of the USA. 2009;**106**:2371-2376

[39] Takayama F, Taki K, Niwa T. Bifidobacterium in gastro-resistant seamless capsule reduces serum levels of indoxyl sulfate in patients on hemodialysis. American Journal of Kidney Diseases. 2003;**41**:S142-S145

[40] Wang IK, Wu YY, Yang YF, Ting IW, Lin CC, Yen TH, et al. The effect of probiotics on serum levels of cytokine and endotoxin in peritoneal dialysis patients: A randomised, double-blind, placebo-controlled trial. Beneficial Microbes. 2015;**6**:423-430

[41] Davani-Davari D, Negahdaripour M, Karimzadeh I, Seifan M, Mohkam M, Masoumi SJ, et al. Prebiotics: Definition, types, sources, mechanisms, and clinical applications. Food. 2019;**8**(3):92. DOI: 10.3390/foods8030092

[42] Duncan SH, Louis P, Thomson JM, Flint HJ. The role of pH in determining the species composition of the human

colonic microbiota. Environmental Microbiology. 2009;**11**(8):2112-2122. DOI: 10.1111/j.1462-2920.2009.01931.x

[43] Guldris SC, Parra EG, Amenós AC. Gut microbiota in chronic kidney disease. Nefrología. 2017;**37**:9-19

[44] Mishima E, Fukuda S, Shima H, Hirayama A, Akiyama Y, Takeuchi Y, et al. Alteration of the intestinal environment by lubiprostone is associated with amelioration of adenine-induced CKD. Journal of the American Society of Nephrology. 2015;**26**:1787-1794

[45] Yamamoto S, Kazama JJ, Omori K, Matsuo K, Takahashi Y, Kawamura K, et al. Continuous reduction of protein-bound uraemic toxins with improved oxidative stress by using the oral charcoal adsorbent AST-120 in haemodialysis patients. Scientific Reports. 2015;**5**:14381

[46] Mishima E, Fukuda S, Kanemitsu Y, Saigusa D, Mukawa C, Asaji K, et al. Canagliflozin reduces plasma uremic toxins and alters the intestinal microbiota composition in a chronic kidney disease mouse model. American Journal of Physiology—Renal Physiology. 2018;**315**:F824-F833

[47] Heerspink HJ, Desai M, Jardine M, Balis D, Meininger G, Perkovic V. Canagliflozin slows progression of renal function decline independently of glycemic effects. Journal of the American Society of Nephrology. 2017;**28**:368-375

[48] Rysz J, Franczyk B, Ławiński J, Olszewski R, Ciałkowska-Rysz A, Gluba-Brzózka A. The impact of CKD on uremic toxins and gut microbiota. Toxins (Basel). 2021;**13**(4):252. DOI: 10.3390/toxins13040252

Chapter 3

Optical Online Monitoring of Uremic Toxins beyond Urea

Fredrik Uhlin and Ivo Fridolin

Abstract

This chapter presents origin and physical basis of the optical method for traditional haemodialysis (HD) dose assessment, accepted as a valid bloodless, robust, automatic, *in situ* and online monitoring technology in clinical praxis. Dialysis dose Kt/V, total removed urea (TRU) and the nutrition parameters PCR, nPCR estimation from ultraviolet (UV) absorbance in the spent dialysate is explained. Since urea, a small water-soluble uremic solute and a surrogate marker for the efficiency of dialysis treatment to clear the blood of toxins and metabolic end products, is not representative for all retained uremic toxins removed with the modern dialysis care, new developments of optical online monitoring of uremic toxins, beyond urea, are discussed. Optical intradialytic monitoring of small-, middle- and protein-bound molecules' removal, exemplified by marker molecules uric acid, beta-2 microglobulin and indoxyl sulphate, is described. A new concept and sensor technology for multi-component uremic toxins' intradialytic optical monitoring of spent dialysate with some clinical examples are introduced. Drug interference studies during the optical dialysis monitoring and future directions in optical monitoring are included. Offered benefits will be more patient-centred, integrated and cost-efficient care, as feedback for clinicians helps to improve and personalize the treatment quality, minimizing costly adverse effects.

Keywords: dialysis dose, dialysis adequacy, fluorescence spectroscopy, haemodialysis, online monitoring, optics, small uremic toxins, middle molecule uremic toxins, protein-bound uremic toxins, ultraviolet absorbance, solute removal, spent dialysate

1. Introduction

The traditional surrogate marker for dialysis dose, urea, which should reflect the clearance of various toxins and metabolic end products is disputed [1]. Removing a sufficient quantity of urea makes it possible to reduce symptoms, morbidity and mortality, and improve quality of life [2]. Urea has over the years been attempted to be measured online in the spent dialysate with different techniques such as enzymatic-, conductivity- and optical sensors. The enzymatic technique measure urea concentrations in the effluent spent dialysate stream, online, using either an ammonium ion (NH4 +) sensor that measures the amount of NH4 + determined directly by an ion-specific electrode or by an electrical potential difference between two electrodes, generated from hydrolysis of urea produces NH4+. A urease membrane catalyzes the chemical reaction when it comes in contact with urea in dialysate [3, 4]. This online technique has disappeared from the market possibly due to cumbersome handling for the staff and high extra costs. There are two still present techniques, first the ionic dialysance method uses a conductivity sensor [5] and is based on the fact that the diffusion coefficients of sodium and urea are similar at 37°C, through a dialysis membrane, therefore sodium dialysance can be used as a marker for urea clearance. The second commercially available technique is the optical method, which will be presented in more detail in this chapter. This technique utilizes the high correlation, in spent dialysate, between urea and UV absorbance at a certain wavelength range, even when urea itself does not absorb UV light [6, 7].

Urea shows a kinetic behavior that is not representative of all retained uremic toxins, including other water-soluble molecules belonging to the group of small molecules. A more comprehensive picture is needed for assessment of uremic solute removal during dialysis involving kinetic profiling and monitoring of the key molecules of all three groups (small-, middle- and protein-bound molecules) of solutes in uremic toxicity [1, 8, 9]. European Renal Best Practice has pointed out that beta-2 microglobulin (β2M) is a potential marker for the middle-size group having a kinetic behavior sufficiently representative of other middle molecules, including peptides of similar size [10, 11]. The protein-bound group, indoxyl sulphate (IS), has received attention because of its link to cardiovascular disease and mortality [12]. Furthermore, analyzing concentrations of these molecules requires today the cumbersome high-performance liquid chromatography (HPLC) method, which, therefore, has limited possibilities to be used in daily clinical practice.

A combined optical online technology utilizing simultaneously both UV absorbance and fluorescence might be a solution for this. This chapter will mainly focus on the latest research and development in that direction and will conclude with the results achieved so far.

2. Optical online monitoring of dialysis dose

2.1 Background of optical dialysis dose monitoring

Optical methods in dialysis dose monitoring started approximately 40 years ago with the development of the HPLC technique, which utilizes UV/Visible (Vis) spectroscopic data for analysis [13–16]. HPLC was utilized for molecule separation and identification of contents in plasma, urine and spent dialysate [17–20]. The "era of uremic toxins search" was born.

Applying standard laboratory photometers to measure solute removal during haemodialysis (HD) was first introduced by Boda and coworkers [21] who demonstrated an exponential decline of UV absorption in spent dialysate at wavelength 210 nm. The introduction of light-fiber optics and the developments of monochromator-detector in the mid-1980s and early-1990s, respectively, entailed near infrared spectroscopy (NIRS) becoming more powerful for scientific research. First, at the end of the 20th century, both UV- and NIRS-techniques were developed forward as practical tools applied for HD dose monitoring.

A Hungarian group published the first report about how UV transmittance of the spent dialysate can be measured at 254 nm, believed to be the best wavelength to monitor the efficacy of HD, [22]. Besides, there was concluded that the hardly diffusible components had a higher elimination rate compared to the removal rate of small, more freely diffusible constituents. Nearly two decades later, a work aiming to monitor the dialysis liquid during HD by UV absorbance was presented by Vasilevski et al. [23]. They also discussed UV extinction as an indicator of nucleic acid metabolism [24]. Almost simultaneously, in 2001, independent studies about online monitoring of solutes in dialysate using UV absorbance were published [6, 25], studying the possibility to monitor removal of different uremic solutes in the spent dialysate, and further firstly describing, as an illustrative example, how to estimate urea Kt/V from UV absorbance. The first clinical study, incorporating the UV-technology with a real clinical application, Kt/V calculation, was reported by Uhlin et al. [7]. A fruitful and exciting collaboration between Uhlin, Fridolin and co-workers within the field of optical dialysis dose monitoring has been followed. During the last decade, in connection with commercialization of the UV-technology for dialysis dose monitoring, new interest has appeared in the optical field. Some works, by the groups from Japan, related to spectroscopic analysis of uremic substances in dialysate have been presented [26, 27] and additionally some papers from St. Petersburg [28]. Validation of a clinical prototype device [29] and the commercially available UV absorbance dialysis dose monitor have been also presented [30]. The UV absorbance method as an alternative method to measure small-solute clearance is mentioned in DOQI clinical practice guideline for haemodialysis adequacy [31]. Moreover, the clinical care guidelines are available to interpret the real-time haemodialysate UV absorbance patterns to optimize solute clearance, troubleshoot problematic absorbance patterns and intervene during an individual treatment as needed [32].

2.2 Overview of optical principles in spectroscopy

Optical dialysis monitoring techniques utilize mostly phenomena described by the optics of biological fluids. Biological fluids include all kinds of fluids made by living organisms like urine, lymph, saliva blood, semen, mucus, gastric juice, aqueous humor, etc. Spent dialysate can also be categorized as a biological fluid derived by filtering the compounds usually less in size than 50,000 Dalton from blood through a dialyzer membrane into the pure dialysate containing water and electrolytes.

From the perspective of optics, biological tissues and fluids can be divided into two large classes: strongly scattering (opaque) tissues and fluids, such as skin, brain, vessel walls, blood, milk lymph and eye sclera, and weakly scattering (transparent) tissues and fluids such as crystalline lens, cornea, vitreous humor, aqueous humor of the front chamber of the eye [33] and spent dialysate. For the second class, the Beer–Lambert law is often applicable [34]. In this section, we will present a short description of the electromagnetic spectrum, some basic principles about photon propagation in biological fluids, Beer–Lambert law and examples of how this could be utilized as a measurement.

2.2.1 Electromagnetic radiation

Electromagnetic (EM) radiation used to be classified by wavelength into radio-, microwave, infrared, visible region, ultraviolet and x- and gamma-rays. The characteristics of EM radiation depend on its wavelength. An illustration of the EM spectrum range is shown in **Figure 1**. Infra-red (IR) is per definition EM radiation with a wavelength range between 760–0.5 mm, Vis 390–770 nm and UV 100–400 nm. The

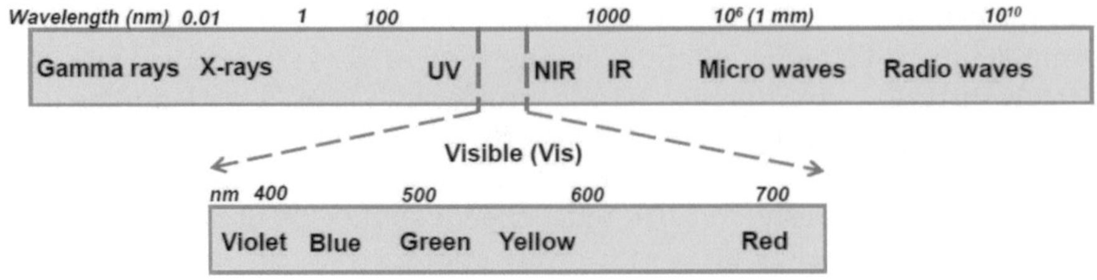

Figure 1.
Illustration of the EM spectrum range.

EM spectrum of UV can be subdivided in a number of ways. The draft ISO standard on determining solar irradiances [35, 36] describes the following ranges relevant to dialysis optical monitoring:

- Ultraviolet A (UVA), long wave 400–315 nm
- Ultraviolet B (UVB), or medium wave 315–280 nm
- Ultraviolet C (UVC), short wave 280–100 nm

"Light" is usually defined as visible EM radiation of the entire EM spectrum where the human eye is sensitive [37–40], but the term light is often extended to adjacent wavelength ranges that the eye cannot detect [40]. Spectroscopy can detect a much wider region of the EM spectrum than the Vis range and a common laboratory spectrophotometer can detect wavelengths from 200 to 2500 nm.

2.2.2 Photon absorption and fluorescence phenomena

Photons that propagate inside a medium can be absorbed by the molecules in the sample.

Absorption: During absorption spectroscopy, an incident photon can be absorbed by a molecule, which leads to the photon energy being converted into an excitation of that molecule's electron cloud. This interaction is sensitive to the internal structure of the molecule since the laws of quantum mechanics only allow for the existence of a limited number of excited states of the electron cloud of any given chemical species. Each of these excited states has a defined energy, the absorption of the photon has to bridge the energy gap between the ground state (lowest energy state) and an allowed excited state of the electron cloud. As a consequence, molecules can be identified by their absorption spectrum, their wavelength-dependent capacity for absorbing photons depends on the energy spacing of the states of their electron cloud. If the frequency of the radiation matches the vibration frequency of the molecule, then radiation will be absorbed, causing a change in the amplitude of molecular vibration [41]. Molecules, which strongly absorb Vis light, appear colored to the human eye and are, therefore, called chromophores, that is "carriers of color".

Fluorescence: In absorption, the signal of molecules in a sample is direct but it can be done with higher sensitivity by using an indirect approach, fluorescence detection. Then the ingoing light will give the absorbing molecules excited states (higher energy) of their electron cloud as described above. From this state, the molecule can shift, "relax", to the electronic ground state by transforming the excess energy into an outgoing emitted light having longer wavelengths than the ingoing light. Different molecules have different emitted spectrums, which being applied during the fluorescence measurements [42].

2.2.3 Beer-Lambert law

The Beer–Lambert law states that the absorbance of light intensity is proportional to the concentration of the substance. This means that the amount of, for example, UV-light absorbed when passing through a cuvette (manufactured by UV-transparent material such as quartz) with spent dialysate, **Figure 2**, is linearly dependent on the concentration c [mol/L] of the absorbing solute, the optical pathlength in (l) [m] (depth of the cuvette) and the extinction coefficient ε $[m^{-1}\,(mol/L)^{-1}]$, even called the molar absorptivity at a certain wavelength [43].

If I_0 is the intensity of the incident light and I is the intensity transmitted light through the medium, the absorbance (A), dimensionless, is Eq. (1):

$$A = \log_{10}\left[\frac{I_0}{I}\right] = \varepsilon \cdot c \cdot l \tag{1}$$

If ε is known for a substance, the absorbance (A) can be calculated by multiplying the path length and the concentration of the substance. If ε is known for a substance and A is obtained from a measurement, it is possible to derive the concentration as Eq. (2):

$$c = \frac{A}{\varepsilon \cdot l} \tag{2}$$

In our case, when the spent dialysate contains several different absorbing compounds, the overall extinction coefficient is the linear sum of the contributions of each compound. However, all the components are not identified and probably there is interference between different substances, which makes it difficult to separate and determine the concentrations of each solute. Absorbance of a solution, obtained by a double beam spectrophotometer, is given by the Lambert–Beer law as [44, 45] Eq. (3):

$$A = \log\frac{I_0}{I_{r+s}} - \log\frac{I_0}{I_r} = \log\frac{I_r}{I_{r+s}} \tag{3}$$

where I_0 is the intensity of incident light from the light source, I_r is the intensity of transmitted light through the reference solution (e.g. pure dialysate) and I_{r+s} is the

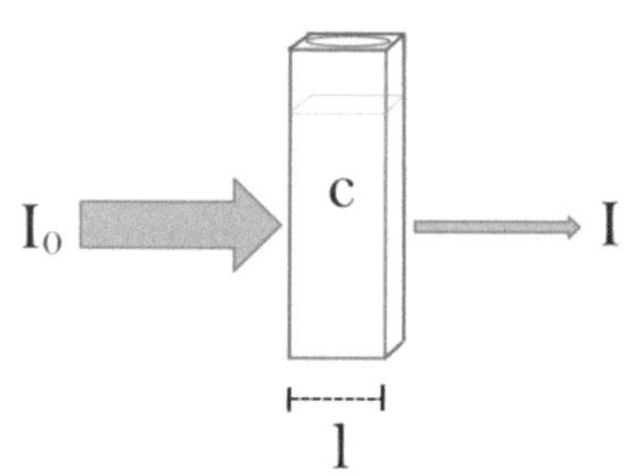

Figure 2.
Cuvette with a sample containing an absorber with concentration, c, ingoing light, I_0, and outgoing light, I, after absorption in the sample when passing through the cuvette with the optical path length, l.

summated intensity of transmitted light through the reference solution mixed with the solution (e.g. pure dialysate + waste products from the blood). The common assumptions to utilize absorbance calculated according to the Beer–Lambert law to determine concentration are: (1) the radiation is monochromatic [34, 43, 46, 47], (2) the irradiating beam is parallel (collimated) across the sample [34, 43], (3) the absorption of radiation for a given species is independent of that of other species [34, 43], (4) only the non-scattered and not-absorbed photons are detected from the medium [40], and (5) the incident radiation and the concentration of the chromophores are not extremely high [46, 48]. The Beer–Lambert law for monochromatic light can be derived by solving a differential equation for a solution with a finite depth containing chromophores and is given in detail in many sources [34, 37, 46]. Analysis of a mixture is based fundamentally on the fact that the absorptions, at each wavelength, of separate components in the mixture are additive, provided that chemical or interfering physical reactions between the components do not occur [43] and the solute concentrations are not very high (not usually found in biological media). In this case, in a medium containing n different absorbing compounds with the concentrations of $c_1 \dots c_n$ [mol/L] and the extinction coefficients of $\varepsilon_1 \dots \varepsilon_n$ $[m^{-1} (mol/L)^{-1}]$, the overall extinction coefficient is simply the linear sum of the contributions of each compound (Eq. (4)):

$$A = \log_{10}\left[\frac{I_0}{I}\right] = (\varepsilon_1 c_1 + \varepsilon_2 c_2 + \dots + \varepsilon_n c_n) l \tag{4}$$

2.2.4 Transmittance and absorbance

The amount of transmitted and absorbed portion of EM radiation in the medium (e.g. in a dialysate sample) can be characterized by the parameter's transmittance T and absorbance A in the spectrophotometer. In order to utilize EM radiation for measurement of constituents in a fluid, the sample is applied in an optical cuvette, **Figure 2**. Through the calibration and measurement procedures, one determines the amount of the ingoing light illuminating the sample symbolized by I_0 and the outgoing light I symbolizing the intensity of the light after passing the sample as the remaining ingoing light is partly absorbed by the sample, **Figure 2**. Having knowledge about those parameters, one can determine transmittance T (Eq. (5)), and absorbance A (Eq. (6)) as:

$$T = \frac{I}{I_0} \Rightarrow \%T = \frac{I}{I_0} \cdot 100\% \tag{5}$$

$$A = -\log T = -\log \frac{I}{I_0} = \log \frac{I_0}{I} \tag{6}$$

3. Dialysis monitoring utilizing UV absorbance technique

Several solutes in spent dialysate identified as uremic toxins by Prof. Vanholder and colleagues in the European Uremic Toxin Work Group (EUTox) have been measured by applying UV absorbance in HPLC technique [49–52]. Currently, two optical techniques for dialysis dose monitoring have been investigated—UV absorbance and NIRS [53, 54]. Other approaches have also been investigated but are more limited so far, for example utilizing the Vis region for measurement. In this chapter, the UV absorbance technique will be discussed that is applied in the commercialized dialysis adequacy monitors ADIMEA [55] and DDM [56]. We will present how clinical parameters based on urea, such as Kt/V, urea reduction ratio (URR), total removed urea (TRU) and protein catabolic rate/protein nitrogen appearance (PCR/PNA), can be estimated optically utilizing UV absorbance.

3.1 Present clinical parameters from optical dialysis dose monitoring

Urea kinetic modeling (UKM), that is where urea is used in differential equations, with the attempt to provide quantitative assessments of dialysis and nutrition adequacy in dialysis patients. The high correlation between urea concentration and UV absorbance values gives consequently the possibility to utilize the UKM equations for UV absorbance similarly. During the UV absorbance and on-line measurements, the pure dialysate was used as the reference, (Eq. (3)) I_r = pure dialysate, and the wavelength was fixed for the entire dialysis. The absorbance baseline level was after the pure flowing dialysate had been stabilized in temperature and conductivity, set to zero when the pure dialysate was flowing through the cuvette prior treatment, see **Figure 3** for the schematic set-up.

3.1.1 Kt/V estimation from UV absorbance

Assuming that urea is distributed in a single pool volume in the body, that urea generation rate and ultrafiltration are negligible during the session and that the ratio K/V remains constant over the dialysis, the following equation holds [57, 58] (Eq. (7)):

$$\mathrm{Kt/V} = -\ln \frac{C_t}{C_0} \tag{7}$$

where C_t is the post and C_0 is the pre-dialysis urea blood concentration, respectively.

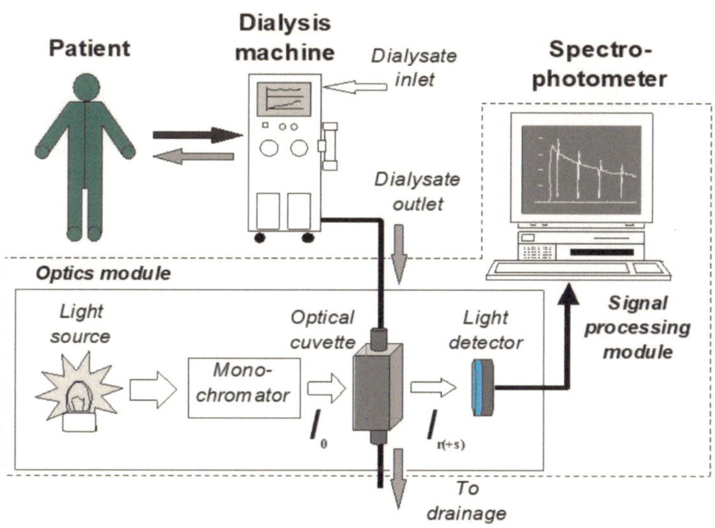

Figure 3.
The schematic set up during the studies. All spent dialysate was also collected in a collection tank to be able to calculate total removal of solutes. [Reprinted from [6]].

From the differential equation, describing urea mass balance during a dialysis session, it can be determined that the average value of the urea clearance (K) in mL/min divided with urea distribution volume in the body (V) in mL (K/V) during a session may be approximated as the slope from the natural logarithm (ln) plot of the urea blood concentration in the blood versus time, S_B. Similarly, but instead of blood urea concentrations, the concentrations of urea in dialysate (S_D) can be used (Eq. (8)). Hence:

$$\mathrm{Kt/V} \approx -S_B\mathrm{T} \approx -S_D\mathrm{T} \tag{8}$$

where T is the dialysis session length in minutes. According to Eq. (8), we obtain Eq. (9):

$$\frac{C_t}{C_0} \approx \exp(-\mathrm{Kt/V}) \approx \exp(S_B\mathrm{T}) \approx \exp(S_D\mathrm{T}) \approx \exp(S_a\mathrm{T}) \tag{9}$$

If the slopes are used instead of the blood urea concentrations. This approximation is equivalent to the equation when two measuring points are used, and the previously mentioned assumptions are fulfilled. This equation would hold strictly if urea obeys fixed volume and single pool kinetics and no urea is generated during the session [59]. In order to calculate Kt/V from the online UV absorbance, the slope of blood or dialysate urea concentration was replaced by the ln slope of the UV absorbance, Sa, see Eq. (9) versus time (Kt/V ≈ – Sa*t, **Figure 4**), [7].

Using the UV absorbance slope values (Sa), **Figure 4**, according to Eq. (9), the Daugirdas-based mono compartmental (single pool, sp) Equation (Eq. (10)) [60]:

$$\mathrm{sp(Kt/V)} = -\ln\left(\frac{C_t}{C_0} - 0.008\frac{\mathrm{T}}{60}\right) + \left(4 - 3.5\frac{C_t}{C_0}\right)\frac{\mathrm{UF}}{\mathrm{BW}} \tag{10}$$

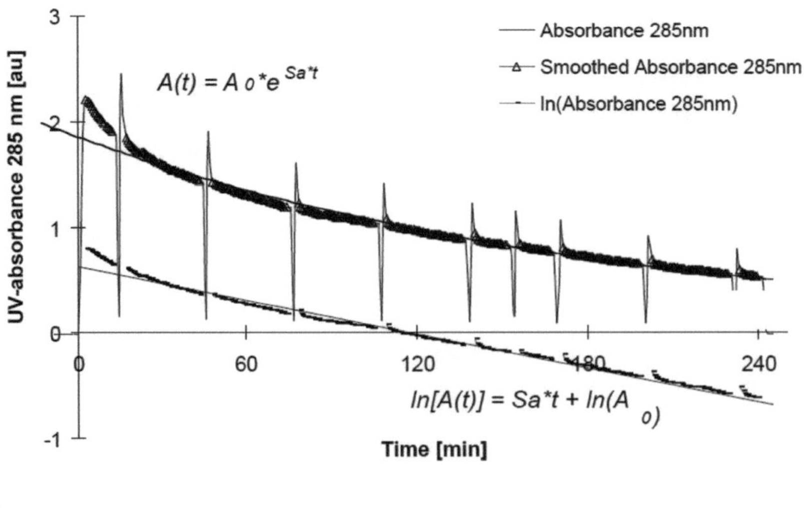

Figure 4.
Online absorbance curve during a single 4 hours HD treatment, where UV absorbance is plotted against time. The corresponding natural logarithmic (ln) fitting line is also shown and used for Kt/V calculation [Reprinted from [7]].

can be written as [7] Eq. (11):

$$sp(Kt/Va) = -\ln\left(\exp(S_aT) - 0.008\frac{T}{60}\right) + (4 - 3.5\exp(S_aT))\frac{UF}{BW} \quad (11)$$

where UF and BW are the ultrafiltration volume in liters (L) and the patient's dry body weight in kg. The equilibrated Kt/V from UV absorbance, eKt/Va, according to the rate adjustment method [60], is predicted from the rate of dialysis (K/V) and the sp(Kt/Va) as Eq. (12):

$$eKt/Va = sp(Kt/Va) - \frac{0.6}{\left(\frac{T}{60}\right)}sp(Kt/Va) + 0.03 \quad (12)$$

The rate adjustment method predicts that the urea rebound is related to the rate of dialysis or dialysis efficiency [61].

3.1.2 Estimation of urea removal using UV absorbance

One way to estimate total removed urea (TRU), assuming that the dialysate flow, Qd(t), is constant and the total UF is known, is to use the following equation (Eq. (13)):

$$TRU(mmol) = \overline{Urea}(Qd \bullet T + UF) \quad (13)$$

where $\overline{Urea}$ in mmol/L is the mean urea concentration in spent dialysate of a particular HD session [62]. For the TRU calculations, Urea = Dtotal can be utilized as reference, where Dtotal is the urea concentration in the collection tank (all spent dialysate from one session), after the end of dialysis. Qd is the rate of the dialysate flow in L/min, T is the dialysis session length in minutes and UF is the total ultrafiltrated volume in L during the session. Under the condition that a good correlation exists between UV absorbance and concentration of urea, it is possible to utilize this relationship. Therefore, in a similar way, TRU may be calculated from the online UV absorbance curve (**Figure 4**) as Eq. (14) [63]:

$$TRUa(mmol) = \left(\alpha \cdot \overline{A} + \beta\right) \cdot (Qd \bullet T + UF) \quad (14)$$

where $\overline{A}$ is the mean of all UV absorbance (A) values from the start to the end of the dialysis. The regression line between the UV absorbance and concentration of urea in spent dialysate from online measurement gives the slope (α) and the intercept (β) inserted in Eq. (14) when determining TRUa from a general model. TRU from the total dialysate collection (TDC), reference, was calculated as Dtotal (mmol/L) multiplied with collected weight (kg), assuming that 1 kg = 1 L of the dialysate [63].

3.1.3 Estimation of nutrition parameters from UV absorbance

High concentration of urea in blood is not necessarily related to a poor dialysis outcome if urea removal is sufficient [64], but also protein-energy malnutrition is frequently present in HD patients. Several studies have suggested that malnutrition is an important risk factor for morbidity and mortality in HD patients [65]. In order to optimize the diet of patients with renal diseases, dietary protein intake has to be controlled. Protein nitrogen appearance (PNA), formerly protein catabolic rate (PCR) [66], is easily obtainable from UKM and in patients who are not markedly catabolic or anabolic, the normalized PNA (nPNA) correlates closely with dietary protein intake [67, 68]. These parameters can be calculated from TRU. The PCR calculation, from TDC and UV absorbance, was based on a theory by Garred et al. (1995), where a calculation of urea removal is expressed as a fraction of the week's urea generation. The fraction varies with the day of the week and was found to be essentially constant among patients on a given day [69]. The amount of urea could, therefore, be approximated by measuring urea concentration from only one of the three treatments and PCR could be calculated as Eq. (15) [63]:

$$nPCRw = Factor_{1,2\text{ or }3}\left(\frac{TRU_{1,2\text{ or }3}}{BW}\right) + 0.17 \tag{15}$$

where TRU 1, 2 or 3 (expressed in grams of urea nitrogen) is the TRU from the first (1), midweek (2) or last dialysis in week (3) and Factor one, two or three is the fractional factor for the corresponding days; factor one = 2.45; two = 2.89 and three = 3.10 [69]. Obligatory loss of dietary protein in stools and via skin shedding represents the constant term 0.17 (g protein/kg body weight/day). BW was used for normalization of PCR (nPCRw). Observe that these fractional factors relay to a treatment schedule of three times a week. More frequent dialysis treatments are common today whereas the factors are not appropriate.

4. Monitoring uremic toxins beyond urea

The fact that urea is considered generally a nontoxic substance and only a marker for uremic retention solutes, and the EUTox has identified several more relevant uremic toxins utilizing optical analysis methods, arise a question connected to further development of optical techniques "Could some of these identified uremic toxins be measured optically on-line?" Of the 90 compounds that have been identified as uremic toxins by the EUTox group [51, 52, 70], we have, from spectroscopic databases, identified 36 to be UV absorbing and among them approximately 25 to be absorbing near 297 nm. In addition to these 90 compounds mentioned as uremic toxins, there are even more solutes in the dialysate that are optically active at 297 nm, which add to the measured UV absorbance signal. Spent dialysate contains numerous different absorbing compounds and concentrations of solutes decline differently during a dialysis session for individuals. The UV absorbance curve may therefore be an individual "clinical print" of the patient's sum of several UV absorbing solutes and therefore a possible parameter for monitoring total solute removal during dialysis. Analyses still remain to find the single solute's individual contribution to the absorbance signal, which is also dependent on which wavelengths are used [71]. Earlier knowledge from the correlation analysis between UV absorbance and a few uremic toxins has shown that it is possible to estimate removal of such solutes, which have a high correlation to UV absorbance. This removal of other uremic retention solutes beyond urea may have stronger impact on dialysis outcomes compared to urea or urea alone.

4.1 Uremic toxins

Uremic toxins used to be divided into three different molecule groups, that is small, water soluble, middle and protein-bound [72], but it needs still to work out their relation to dialysis efficacy and what roles different molecules will have in the development of uremia and which dialysis techniques are best at reducing the elevated levels of these [73]. Proposal for a new classification system of uremic solutes rationale has been made [74]. Declined uremic toxin clearance due to low GFR is not the only cause of toxin accumulation in kidney failure. Excessive production of cytokines and soluble receptors due to local tissue inflammation is a major contributor to the middle molecule accumulation [75], and gut dysbiosis generates a broad spectrum of uremic toxins [76]. Thus, a broader view of uremic solutes that goes beyond simply retention with poor GFR is needed. Recent data regarding the origin of uremic toxins, and the new development of HD methods and new membranes with the ability to clear uremic toxins with specific characteristics, or by using drugs/molecules to facilitate the shift from bound fraction to free fraction [77], have led to propose a new classification beyond the classic physicochemical classification. A study by Vanholder et al. (2018) presents a ranking score list of uremic toxins with known toxicity according to experimental and clinical studies [78], **Table 1** shows the highest- and second-highest evidence-scored uremic toxins.

The uremic toxins with the optical monitoring capacity referred to further in this chapter are marked in underline. AGEs and IAA are in italics as the potential targets for the optical monitoring in the future, **Table 1**.

Highest evidence score	Second highest evidence score
p-cresyl sulfate	*Advanced glycation end products (AGEs)*
β_2-microglobulin	Indoxyl sulfate
Asymmetric dimethyl arginine	Uric acid
Carbamylated compounds	Ghrelin
Fibroblast growth factor-23	*Indole acetic acid (IAA)*
IL-6	Parathyroid hormone
TNF_α	Phenyl acetic acid
Symmetric dimethyl arginine	Trimethyl methylamine-N-oxide
	Retinol binding protein
	Endothelin
	Immunoglobulin light chains
	IL-1β
	IL-8
	Neuropeptide Y
	Lipids and lipoprotein

Table 1.
Uremic toxins with the highest toxicity evidence score (modified from Vanholder et al. 2018) [78].

4.1.1 Optical intradialytic monitoring of small water-soluble molecules' removal

Uric acid, like urea, a representative molecule from the small group of uremic toxins, has been shown to have a high absorption of UV in the wavelength region 280–310 nm (also a peak around 230–240 nm), **Figure 5a**. As a consequence, we have been able to show that it is possible to estimate the total removal of uric acid during dialysis

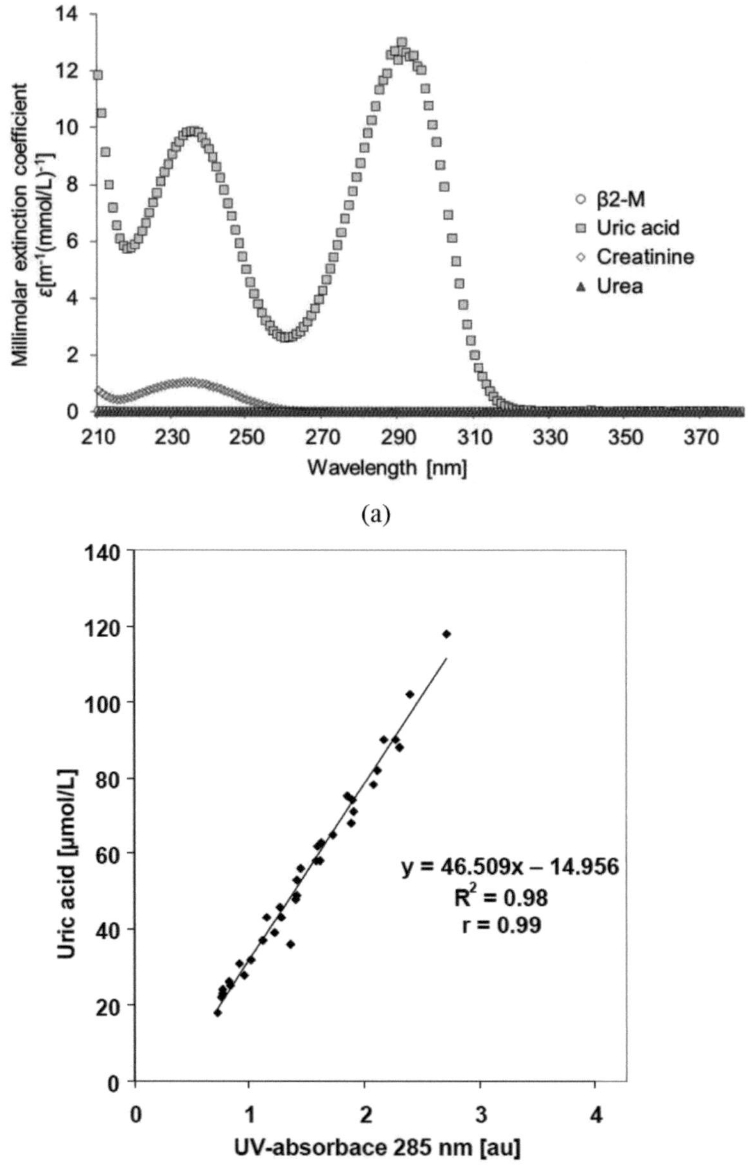

Figure 5.
(a) The molar absorptivity for four solutes, β2M, uric acid, creatinine and urea in 24 HDF sessions. (b) An example of the regression line between concentration of uric acid and UV-absorbance [Figure 5a, reprinted from [86]].

[79, 80] and a multi-wavelength and processed signal approach can provide even more accurate results [81]. **Figure 5b** shows an example of the best-fit regression equation of uric acid vs. UV absorbance in spent dialysate at wavelength 285 nm during four dialysis sessions in the same patient, showing a high correlation of r = 0.99.

Earlier research has demonstrated potential of intradialytic optical monitoring to estimate the removal of low molecular weight uremic solutes other than uric acid as urea [53] and creatinine [82] with their clinical implications. Furthermore, optical monitoring of low molecule weight uremic solutes removal by HD, assessed via the marker molecule urea-related dialysis adequacy parameters, has become a worldwide practice [55, 56, 83]. A possibility for optical monitoring of phosphate and calcium elimination during dialysis has also been presented [84, 85].

4.1.2 Optical intradialytic monitoring of middle molecules' removal

Using UV absorbance alone to estimate β2M does not appear to be optimal even a high correlation between UV absorbance and β2M in spent dialysate can be achieved for HDF but not for HD [86]. Instead, fluorescence spectra could be a better alternative [87] as it is possible to detect the fluorescence of advanced glycation end products (AGE) modified β2M in spent dialysate [88, 89]. However, the measuring system needs high selectivity and sensitivity for detection due to low contribution of AGE modified β2M to overall fluorescence [89]. The best correlation between the fluorescence of spent dialysate and the concentration of β2M in spent dialysate was found in the wavelength region Ex350–370/Em500–555 nm, with the coefficient of determination R^2 up to 0.859, **Figure 6a**.

A multiwavelength fluorescence approach can yield a high correlation of up to 0.958 between laboratory and optically estimated β2M concentrations in spent dialysate. The main contributors to the optical signal of the middle molecule (MM) fraction were provisionally identified as tryptophan (Trp) in small peptides and proteins and AGEs [90]. **Figure 6b** visualize the good agreement between β2M concentrations analyzed in laboratory vs. those predicted by an optical model during 29 four-hour HDF sessions.

4.1.3 Optical intradialytic monitoring of protein-bound molecules' removal

Recent studies have presented that quantification of indoxyl sulphate (IS) in the spent dialysate using fluorescence spectra is possible [91, 92]. **Figure** 7 shows an example of a HPLC chromatogram of a spent dialysate sample taken 10 min after the start of HD, where the fluorescence was recorded at Ex: 280 nm and Em: 360 nm. In total, 12 clearly resolved chromatographic peaks of fluorophoric compounds were detected in most (82%) of the spent dialysate samples during the HPLC analysis collected at different time moments in the dialysis [92]. Of these, five peaks had a major importance in all samples (peaks no 6, 8, 9, 11 and 12), and six of these 12 peaks were identified as Trp and their metabolites of indole derivates: indoxyl glucuronide (IGluc), IS, 5-hydroxy-indole-3-acetic acid, indole acetyl glutamine (IaG) and indole acetic acid (IAA) [92]. IS is one of the main fluorophores in these measuring conditions (**Figure** 7, peak 9) [92]. This is in agreement with the earlier studies, where IS has been found as a main contributor to the fluorescence in uremic fluids [93, 94].

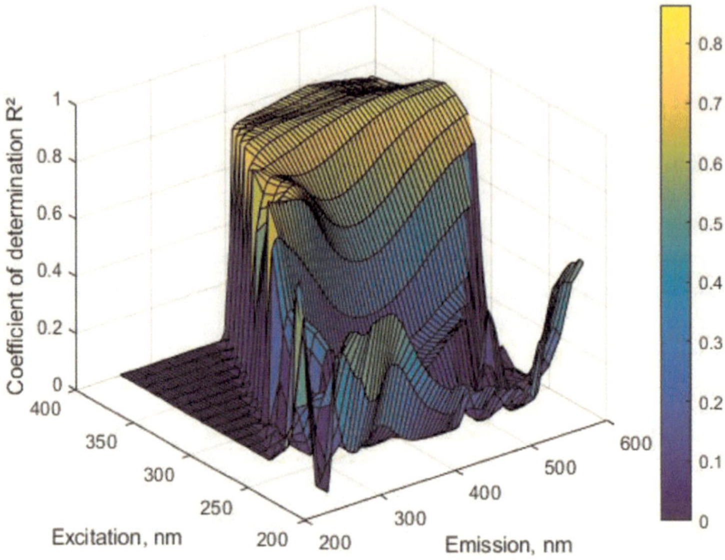

(a)

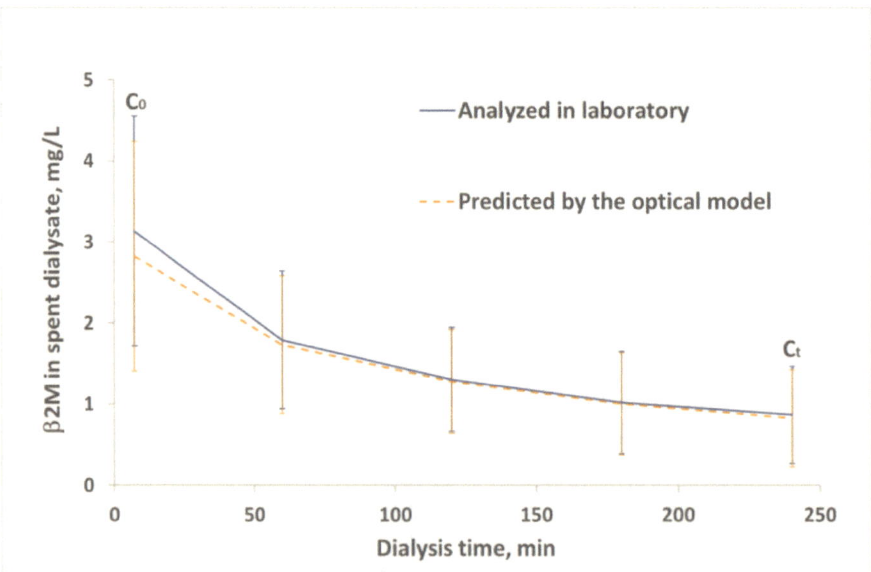

(b)

Figure 6.
a. Wavelength dependence of the correlation between fluorescence intensity and concentration of β2M in spent dialysate for HDF modalities (N = 375). b. Time-series of changing β2M concentration (mean ± SD) in the spent dialysate during HDF dialysis sessions (N = 29) for patients of the validation set [Reprinted from [90]].

4.2 Multi-component uremic toxins' intradialytic optical monitoring of spent dialysate

Several *in vitro* and online studies towards optical multi-component uremic toxins' monitoring have been published by our group during the last 10 years [9, 95–98]

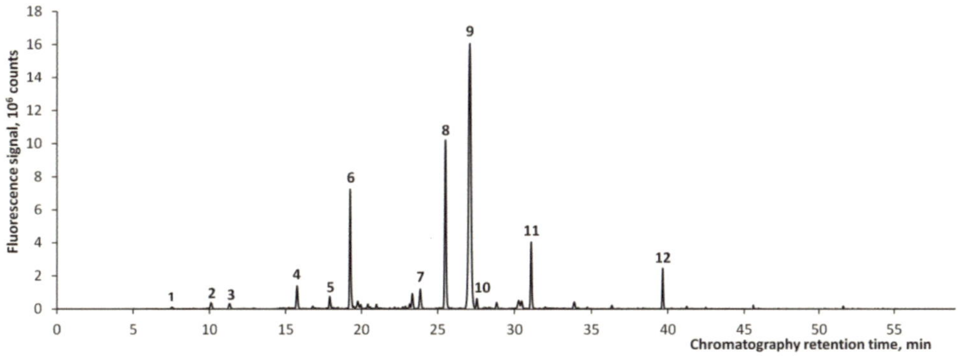

Figure 7.
Example of a chromatogram of a spent dialysate sample, where peak 9 is indoxyl sulphate. [Reprinted from [92]].

and by a group from Taiwan [99]. The studies demonstrate that optical dialysis monitoring, based on UV absorbance and fluorescence of spent dialysate, can simultaneously reveal removal patterns of, for example, urea, β2M and IS during various dialysis treatment modalities without any blood or dialysate sampling, **Figure 8**.

A good agreement between chemically and optically estimated solute removal parameters, RR and total removed solute, was achieved. Dialysis modality did not affect the accuracy of optical method, taking into account that β2M was excluded from the analysis in the case of dialysis with low-flux dialyzer [9]. **Figure 9** shows the agreement in RR (%) for urea, β2M and IS between measurements from laboratory and the developed online optical dialysis adequacy sensor (OLDIAS).

4.2.1 Drug interference during the optical dialysis monitoring in spent dialysate

There have been indications that the administration of some drug chromophores, for example paracetamol (Par), to dialysis patients could disturb the accuracy of the

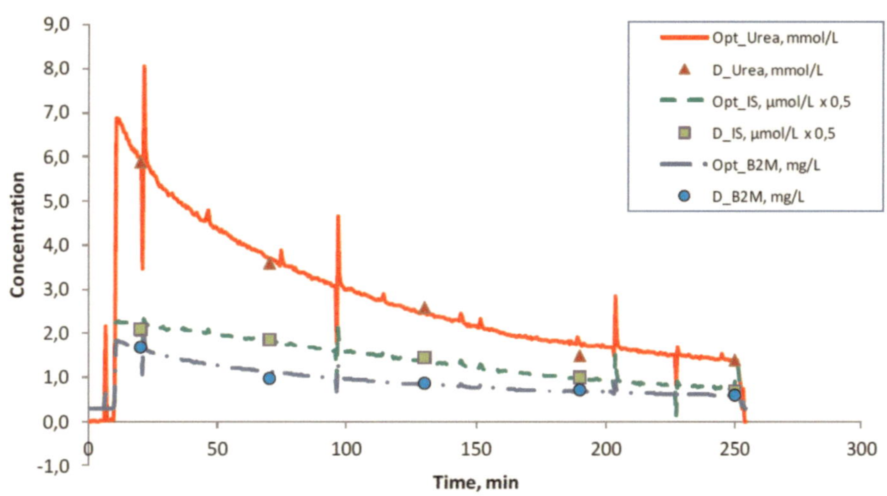

Figure 8.
An example representing real-time concentration profiles for urea, β2M (B2M) and IS during a single dialysis from optical measurements in the spent dialysate in parallel with the discrete concentration values estimated from the laboratory analyses of spent dialysate samples at different time moments.

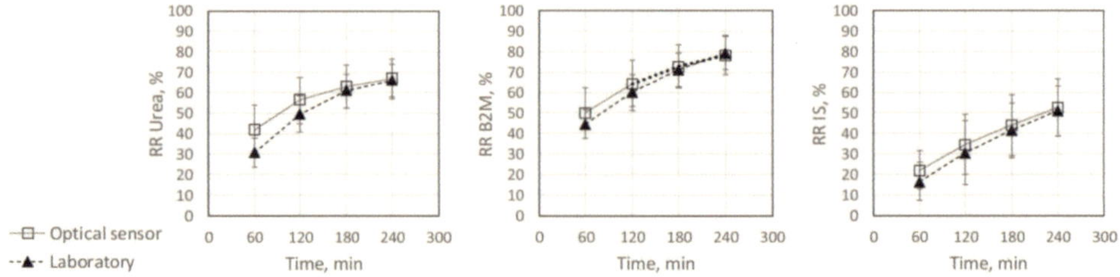

Figure 9.
A comparison presenting the agreement in RR for urea (Urea), β2M (B2M) and indoxyl sulphate (IS) between measurements from laboratory and the online optical dialysis adequacy sensor (OLDIAS).

optical methods since a noteworthy contribution of Par and its metabolites to the total UV absorbance was determined at three wavelengths 210, 254 and 280 nm [100], where the latter is used in the commercial monitor [56]. Adoberg et al. confirmed that the administration of Par in large amounts increased the UV absorbance of spent dialysate, which can result in overestimation of concentration and the RR of uric acid (UA) when evaluated by UV absorbance of spent dialysate, using the UV region that overlaps with the Par-absorption spectrum [101]. At the same time, the correlation between the IS concentration and fluorescence in the spent dialysate is not affected by Par administration to dialysis patients, neither is the optical assessment of the RR of IS on the basis of the fluorescence of spent dialysate. **Figure 10** illustrates a representative chromatogram of the spent dialysate of a patient with high Par intake (twice 1 g of Par before dialysis, 1 g during the dialysis session and four times 1 g on the previous day) and the UV absorbance spectra of Par, Par metabolites and UA peaks on the insert.

These limitations could be overcome by using multiparametric optical models that incorporate several UV wavelengths in order to evaluate the removal of UA, and also urea, or using the UV region, such as 295 nm, to minimize the influence of Par.

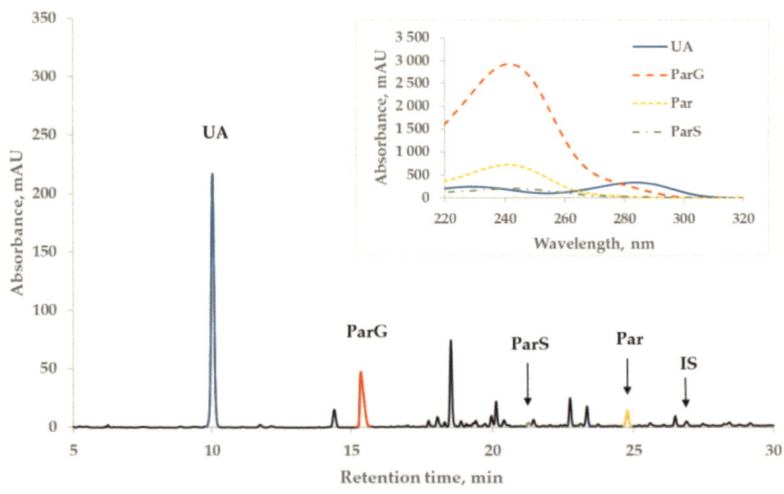

Figure 10.
Characteristic HPLC UV 295 nm chromatogram of spent dialysate of one patient with high Par intake. Insert: UV-absorbance spectra of peaks of uric acid (UA), paracetamol glucuronide (ParG), paracetamol (Par), paracetamol sulphate (ParS), and indoxyl sulphate (IS) [Reprinted from [101]].

Conventionally prescribed drugs in connection with dialysis treatment did not interfere with the optical monitoring of the treatment [101].

4.2.2 Future directions in optical monitoring

The future vision of the dialysis optical monitoring technology is moving towards the ability to estimate efficacy measures of several important uremic toxins, for example, **Figure 8** that are linked to morbidity and survival for dialysis patients.

Attempts of optical intradialytic monitoring of AGE's have also been carried out within our group, showing no difference between average of free pentosidine concentrations in the spent dialysate measured by HPLC and models, developed from the full fluorescence spectra [102]. Tryptophan, which originates uremic toxins that contribute to end-stage kidney disease (ESKD) patient outcomes, may also be a target for future monitoring. Paats et al. evaluated serum levels and removal during HD and haemodiafiltration (HDF) of tryptophan and tryptophan-derived uremic toxins, indoxyl sulphate (IS) and indole acetic acid (IAA), in ESKD patients in different dialysis treatment settings [103]. High-efficiency HDF resulted in 80% higher Trp losses than conventional low-flux dialysis, despite similar neutral Trp RR values. In conclusion, serum Trp concentrations and RR behave differently from uremic solutes IS, IAA and urea and Trp RR did not reflect dialysis Trp losses. Conventional low-flux dialysis may not adequately clear Trp-related uremic toxins while high-efficiency HDF increased Trp losses [103]. Furthermore, by adding chemical displacers, combining ibuprofen and furosemide, during HDF, the removal of protein-bound uremic toxins can be enhanced [104, 105].

Finally, the technology will be integrated into the dialysis machines of the future for simple handling and easy monitoring over time, **Figure 11**.

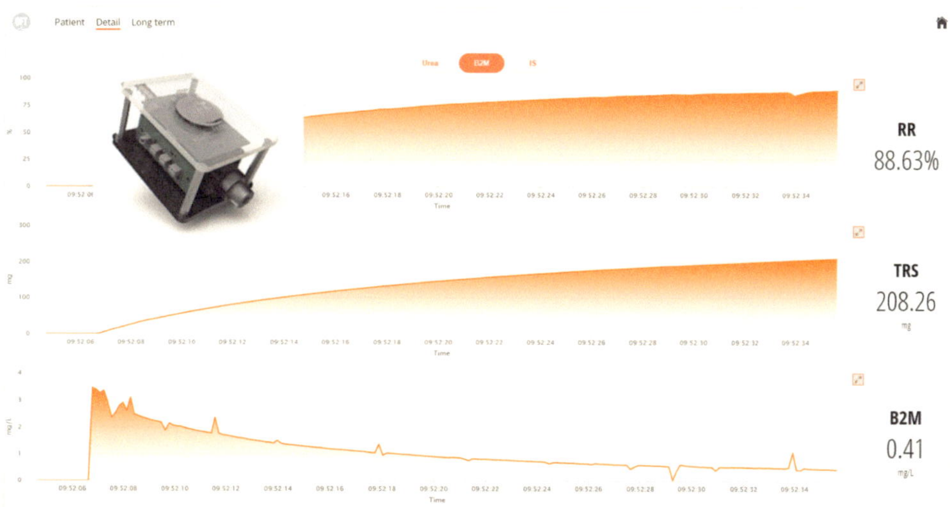

Figure 11.
An example of a future display on the dialysis machine where multiple performance measures (removal ratio, total removed amount, Kt/V) for β2M (B2M) (Courtesy of Optofluid Technologies OÜ, Estonia, with permission).

5. Conclusion

Uremia occurs due to retention of a variety of substances with different properties. Historically, we have had one marker, urea, to describe the total uremic environment in dialysis patients. There is a need to follow a wider spectrum of uremic toxins that are more strongly linked to morbidity and survival than urea alone. Our ambition with this research, using combined optical methods, is to be able to monitor several important uremic toxins online in the future. Patients will benefit from more patient-centred, integrated and cost-efficient care, as feedback for clinicians helps to improve and personalize the treatment quality, minimizing costly adverse effects. Feedback to patients helps to integrate patients into their own treatment, increasing patients' compliance and well-being.

Acknowledgements

Thanks to all colleagues who have been involved in the projects: Risto Tanner, Merike Luman, Jana Holmar, Jürgen Arund, Sigrid Kalle, Ruth Tomson, Rain Ferenets, Joosep Paats, Kai Lauri, Annika Adoberg, Liisi Leis, Mårten Segelmark, Anders Fernström, Kristjan Pilt, Deniss Karai, Micael Gylling and Kelly Stjernfelt, Martin Magnusson, Lars-Göran Lindberg.

Author details

Fredrik Uhlin[1,2]* and Ivo Fridolin[2]

1 Department of Nephrology and Department of Health, Medicine and Caring Sciences, Linköping University, Linköping, Sweden

2 Department of Health Technologies, Tallinn University of Technology (TalTech), Tallinn, Estonia

*Address all correspondence to: fredrik.uhlin@regionostergotland.se

References

[1] Vanholder R, Glorieux G, Eloot S. Once upon a time in dialysis: The last days of Kt/V? Kidney International. 2015;**88**:460-465. DOI: 10.1038/ki.2015.155

[2] Sehgal AR, Leon JB, Siminoff LA, Singer ME, Bunosky LM, Cebul RD. Improving the quality of hemodialysis treatment. A community-based randomized controlled trial to overcome patient-specific barriers. Journal of the American Medical Association. 2002; **287**:1961-1967. DOI: 10.1001/jama.287.15.1961

[3] Jurkiewicz M, Solé S, Almirall J, García M, Alegret S, Martínez-Fàbregas E. Validation of an automatic urea analyzer used in the continuous monitoring of hemodialysis parameters. The Analyst. 1996;**121**:959-963. DOI: 10.1039/an9962100959

[4] Canaud B, Bosc JY, Leblanc M, Vaussenat F, Leray-Moragues H, Garred LJ, et al. On-line dialysis quantification in acutely ill patients: Preliminary clinical experience with a multipurpose urea sensor monitoring device. ASAIO Journal. 1998;**44**:184-190. DOI: 10.1097/00002480-199805000-00012

[5] Polaschegg HD. Automatic, noninvasive intradialytic clearance measurement. The International Journal of Artificial Organs. 1993;**16**:185-191

[6] Fridolin I, Magnusson M, Lindberg LG. On-line monitoring of solutes in dialysate using absorption of ultraviolet radiation: Technique description. The International Journal of Artificial Organs. 2002;**25**:748-761. DOI: 10.1177/039139880202500802

[7] Uhlin F, Fridolin I, Lindberg LG, Magnusson M. Estimation of delivered dialysis dose by on-line monitoring of the ultraviolet absorbance in the spent dialysate. American Journal of Kidney Diseases. 2003;**41**:1026-1036. DOI: 10.1016/s0272-6386(03)00200-2

[8] Eloot S, Schneditz D, Cornelis T, Van Biesen W, Glorieux G, Dhondt A, et al. Protein-bound uremic toxin profiling as a tool to optimize hemodialysis. PLoS One. 2016;**11**:e0147159. DOI: 10.1371/journal.pone.0147159

[9] Lauri K, Arund J, Holmar J, Tanner R, Kalle S, Luman M, et al. Removal of urea, β2-microglobulin, and indoxyl sulfate assessed by absorbance and fluorescence in the spent dialysate during hemodialysis. ASAIO Journal. 2020;**66**:698-705. DOI: 10.1097/MAT.0000000000001058

[10] Tattersall J, Martin-Malo A, Pedrini L, Basci A, Canaud B, Fouque D, et al. EBPG guideline on dialysis strategies. Nephrology Dialysis Transplantation. 2007;**22**(Suppl. 2):ii5-i21. DOI: 10.1093/ndt/gfm022

[11] Pedrini L, Kessler M, Canaud B, Tattersali J, Ter Wee P, Vanholder R, et al. European Best Practice Guidelines Expert Group on Hemodialysis, European Renal Association. Section II. Haemodialysis adequacy. Nephrol Dial Transplant. 2002;**17**(Suppl 7):16-31. PMID: 12386211

[12] Vanholder R, Schepers E, Pletinck A, Nagler EV, Glorieux G. The uremic toxicity of indoxyl sulfate and p-cresyl sulfate: A systematic review. Journal of the American Society of Nephrology. 2014;**25**:1897-1907. DOI: 10.1681/ASN.2013101062

[13] Gordon A, Berström J, Fürst P, Zimmerman L. Separation and

characterization of uremic metabolites in biologic fluids: A screening approach to the definition of uremic toxins. Kidney International Supplement. 1975; **2**:45-51

[14] Asaba H, Fürst P, Oulés R, Yahiel V, Zimmerman L, Bergström J. The effect of hemodialysis on endogenous middle molecules in uremic patients. Clinical Nephrology. 1979;**11**:257-266

[15] Schoots AC, Homan HR, Gladdines MM, Cramers CA, de Smet R, Ringoir SM. Screening of UV-absorbing solutes in uremic serum by reversed phase HPLC–Change of blood levels in different therapies. Clinica Chimica Acta. 1985;**146**:37-51. DOI: 10.1016/0009-8981(85)90122-6

[16] Gróf J, Menyhárt J. Molecular weight distribution, diffusibility and comparability of middle molecular fractions prepared from normal and uremic sera by different fractionation procedures. Nephron. 1982;**30**:60-67. DOI: 10.1159/000182434

[17] Brunner H, Mann H. Combination of conventional and high-performance liquid chromatographic techniques for the isolation of so-called "uraemic toxins". Journal of Chromatography. 1984;**297**:405-416. DOI: 10.1016/s0021-9673(01)89062-2

[18] Mabuchi H, Nakahashi H. Determination of 3-carboxy-4-methyl-5-propyl-2-furanpropanoic acid, a major endogenous ligand substance in uremic serum, by high-performance liquid chromatography with ultraviolet detection. Journal of Chromatography. 1987;**415**:110-117. DOI: 10.1016/s0378-4347(00)83197-7

[19] Vanholder RC, De Smet RV, Ringoir SM. Assessment of urea and other uremic markers for quantification of dialysis efficacy. Clinical Chemistry. 1992;**38**:1429-1436

[20] Vanholder R, De Smet R, Jacobs V, Van Landschoot N, Waterloos MA, et al. Uraemic toxic retention solutes depress polymorphonuclear response to phagocytosis. Nephrology, Dialysis, Transplantation. 1994;**9**:1271-1278

[21] Boda D, Gál G, Eck E, Kiss E. Ultraviolet spectrophotomerty studies of serum dialysate from patients with long term intermittent artificial kidney treatment. Zeitschrift für Urologie und Nephrologie. 1977;**70**:345-349

[22] Gál G, Gróf J. Continuous UV photometric monitoring of the efficiency of hemodialysis. The International Journal of Artificial Organs. 1980;**3**: 338-341

[23] Vasilevski AM, Kornilov NV. Monitoring the dialysis liquid during hemodialysis from the extinction spectra in the UV region. Journal of Optical Technology. 1999;**66**:692

[24] Vasilevsky AM, Konoplyov GA. Peculiar character of dialyzate ultraviolet extinction spectra as an indicator of nucleic acid metabolism in humans. Journal of Biomedical Optics. 2005;**10**: 44026. DOI: 10.1117/1.1953268

[25] Fridolin I, Magnusson M, Lindberg LG. Measurement of solutes in dialysate using UV absorption. In: Proceedings of the International Society for Optical Engineering Conference. San Jose. USA: Society of Photo-Optical Instrumentation Engineers (SPIE); 2001. DOI: 10.1117/12.429345

[26] Umimoto K, Tatsumi Y, Kanaya H, Jokei K. Analysis of uremic substances in dialysate by visible ultraviolet spectroscopy. In: Magjarevic R,

Nagel JH, editors. World Congress on Medical Physics and Biomedical Engineering. IFMBE Proceedings. Berlin: Springer; 2006. DOI: 10.1007/978-3-540-36841-0_810

[27] Umimoto K, Kanaya Y, Kawanishi H, Kawai N. Measuring of uremic substances in dialysate by visible ultraviolet spectroscopy. In: Dössel O, Schlegel WC, editors. World Congress on Medical Physics and Biomedical Engineering, September 7 - 12, 2009, Munich, Germany. IFMBE Proceedings. Vol 25/7. Berlin, Heidelberg: Springer; 2009. DOI: 10.1007/978-3-642-03885-3_12

[28] Vasilevskiy AM, Konoplev GA. Polycomponental monitoring of process of effluent dialyzate by a method of uf of spectrometry. Biotekhnosfera. 2009. Available from: https://scholar.google.com/scholar?cluster=6506178806057926161 [Accessed: 2020-2112-23]

[29] Luman M, Jerotskaja J, Lauri K, Fridolin I. Dialysis dose and nutrition assessment by optical on-line dialysis adequacy monitor. Clinical Nephrology. 2009;**72**:303-311. DOI: 10.5414/cnp72303

[30] Castellarnau A, Werner M, Günthner R, Jakob M. Real-time Kt/V determination by ultraviolet absorbance in spent dialysate: Technique validation. Kidney International. 2010;**78**:920-925. DOI: 10.1038/ki.2010.216

[31] National Kidney Foundation. KDOQI clinical practice guideline for hemodialysis adequacy: 2015 update. American Journal of Kidney Diseases. 2015;**66**:884-930. DOI: 10.1053/j.ajkd.2015.07.015

[32] Ross EA, Paugh-Miller JL, Nappo RW. Interventions to improve hemodialysis adequacy: Protocols based on real-time monitoring of dialysate solute clearance. Clinical Kidney Journal. 2018;**11**:394-399. DOI: 10.1093/ckj/sfx110

[33] Tuchin VV. Tissue Optics: Light Scattering Methods and Instruments for Medical Diagnosis. Bellingham: SPIE Press; 2007. DOI: 10.1117/3.684093

[34] Regan JD, Parrish JA. The Science of Photomedicine. New York: Plenum Press; 1982. p. 658. DOI: 10.1007/978-1-4684-8312-3

[35] ISO21348 Process for determining solar irradiances. 2007. Available from: https://cdn.standards.iteh.ai/samples/39911/7088f5099b2343c3810f06b6ca9bc35b/ISO-21348-2007.pdf [Accessed 2022-2112-01]

[36] Van de Hulst HC. Multiple Light Scattering Tables, Formulas and Applications. New York: Academic Press; 1980. DOI: 10.1016/B978-0-12-710701-1.X5001-0

[37] Sliney DH, Wolbarsht M. Safety with Lasers and Other Optical Sources. New York: Plenum Press; 1980

[38] Judy MM. Biomedical lasers. In: Bronzino JD, editor. The Biomedical Engineering Handbook. Boca Raton, FL: CRC Press; 1995. pp. 1334-1345

[39] Saleh BEA, Teich MC. Fundamentals of Photonics. New York: John Wiley & Sons, Inc.; 1991

[40] Welch AJ, van Gemert MJC, Star WM, Wilson BC. Definitions and overview of tissue optics. In: Welch AJ, van Gemert MJC, editors. Optical-Thermal Response of Laser-Irradiated Tissue. New York: Plenum Press; 1995. pp. 15–46

[41] Lajunen LHJ, Perämäki P. Spectrochemical Analysis by Atomic

Absorption and Emission. Wakefield: The Royal Society of Chemistry. Charlesworth Group; 2004. pp. 1-342. DOI: 10.1039/9781847551900

[42] Lakowicz JR. Principles of Fluorescence Spectroscopy. 3rd ed. New York: Springer Science + Business Media, LLC; 2006. pp. 1-673. DOI: 10.1007/978-0-387-46312-4

[43] Glasser O. Medical Physics. Chicago: The Year Book Inc.; 1961

[44] Hahn B, Vlastelica DL, Snyder LR, Furda J, Rao KJ. Polychromatic analysis: New applications of an old technique. Clinical Chemistry. 1979;**25**: 951-959

[45] Zwart A, Buursma A, van Kampen EJ, Zijlstra WG. Multicomponent analysis of hemoglobin derivatives with reversed-optics spectrophotometer. Clinical Chemistry. 1984;**30**:373-379

[46] Mann CK, Vickers TJ, Gulick WM. Ultraviolet–visible absorption spectroscopy. In: Instrumental Analysis. New York: Harper & Row; 1974. pp. 427-452

[47] Björn LO. Optiska och elektriska analysmetoder. Stockholm: Almqvist & Wiksell; 1965

[48] Togawa T, Tamura T, Öberg PÅ. Biomedical Transducers and Instruments. New York: CRC Press; 1997

[49] Vanholder R, Van Laecke S, Glorieux G. What is new in uremic toxicity? Pediatric Nephrology. 2008;**23**: 1211-1221. DOI: 10.1007/s00467-008-0762-9

[50] Vanholder RC, De Smet R, Lameire NH. Uremic toxicity. In: Hörl WH, Koch KM, Lindsay RM, Ronco C, Winchester JF, editors. Replacement of Renal Function by Dialysis. Dordrecht: Springer; 2004. DOI: 10.1007/978-1-4020-2275-3_2

[51] Vanholder R, De Smet R, Glorieux G, Argilés A, Baurmeister U, Brunet P, et al. European uremic toxin work group (EUTox). Review on uremic toxins: Classification, concentration, and interindividual variability. Kidney International. 2003;**63**:1934-1943. DOI: 10.1046/j.1523-1755.2003.00924.x

[52] Vanholder R, Glorieux G, De Smet R, Lameire N. European uremic toxin work group. New insights in uremic toxins. Kidney International. Supplement. 2003; **84**:S6-S10. DOI: 10.1046/j.1523-1755.63.s84.43.x

[53] Uhlin F, Fridolin I, Magnusson M, Lindberg LG. Dialysis dose (Kt/V) and clearance variation sensitivity using measurement of ultraviolet-absorbance (on-line), blood urea, dialysate urea and ionic dialysance. Nephrology, Dialysis, Transplantation. 2006;**21**:2225-2231. DOI: 10.1093/ndt/gfl147

[54] Olesberg JT, Arnold MA, Flanigan MJ. Online measurement of urea concentration in spent dialysate during hemodialysis. Clinical Chemistry. 2004;**50**:175-181. DOI: 10.1373/clinchem.2003.025569

[55] Adimea Real-Time Monitoring Process. Available from: https://www.bbraun.com/content/dam/catalog/bbraun/bbraunProductCatalog/S/AEM2015/en-01/b3/adimea.pdf. [Accessed: 2020-2112-23]

[56] Kt/v Measurement. Dialysis dose monitor measuring the delivered dialysis dose. Available online: http://nikkisomedical.com/wp-content/uploads/2017/06/DDM_english_2013-03_vers04.pdf. [Accessed: 2020-12-23]

[57] Barth RH. Direct calculation of KT/V. A simplified approach to monitoring of hemodialysis. Nephron. 1988;**50**:191-195. DOI: 10.1159/000185156

[58] Gotch FA, Sargent JA. A mechanistic analysis of the National Cooperative Dialysis Study (NCDS). Kidney International. 1985;**28**:526-534. DOI: 10.1038/ki.1985.160

[59] Gotch FA, Keen ML. Care of the patient on hemodialysis. In: Cogan MG, Schoenfeld P, editors. Introduction to Dialysis. 2nd ed. New York: Churchill Livingstone Inc.; 1991. pp. 101-176

[60] Daugirdas JT. Simplified equations for monitoring Kt/V, PCRn, eKt/V, and ePCRn. Advances in Renal Replacement Therapy. 1995;**2**:295-304. DOI: 10.1016/s1073-4449(12)80028-8

[61] Daugirdas JT, Depner TA, Gotch FA, Greene T, Keshaviah P, Levin NW, et al. Comparison of methods to predict equilibrated Kt/V in the HEMO pilot study. Kidney International. 1997;**52**:1395-1405. DOI: 10.1038/ki.1997.467

[62] Raj DS, Tobe S, Saiphoo C, Manuel MA. Quantitating dialysis using two dialysate samples: A simple, practical and accurate approach for evaluating urea kinetics. The International Journal of Artificial Organs. 1997;**20**:422-427

[63] Uhlin F, Fridolin I, Lindberg LG, Magnusson M. Estimating total urea removal and protein catabolic rate by monitoring UV absorbance in spent dialysate. Nephrology, Dialysis, Transplantation. 2005;**20**:2458-2464. DOI: 10.1093/ndt/gfi026

[64] Blumenkrantz MJ, Kopple JD, Moran JK, Coburn JW. Metabolic balance studies and dietary protein requirements in patients undergoing continuous ambulatory peritoneal dialysis. Kidney International. 1982;**21**:849-861. DOI: 10.1038/ki.1982.109

[65] Lindsay RM, Heidenheim AP, Spanner E, Kortas C, Blake PG. Adequacy of hemodialysis and nutrition–Important determinants of morbidity and mortality. Kidney International. Supplement. 1994;**44**:S85-S91

[66] Kooman J, Basci A, Pizzarelli F, Canaud B, Haage P, Fouque D, et al. EBPG guideline on haemodynamic instability. Nephrology, Dialysis, Transplantation. 2007;**22**(Suppl. 2):ii22-ii44. DOI: 10.1093/ndt/gfm019

[67] Flanigan MJ, Lim VS, Redlin J. The significance of protein intake and catabolism. Advances in Renal Replacement Therapy. 1995;**2**:330-340. DOI: 10.1016/s1073-4449(12)80031-8

[68] Keane WF, Collins AJ. Influence of co-morbidity on mortality and morbidity in patients treated with hemodialysis. American Journal of Kidney Diseases. 1994;**24**:1010-1018. DOI: 10.1016/s0272-6386(12)81076-6

[69] Garred LJ, Canaud B, Argiles A, Flavier JL, Mion C. Protein catabolic rate determination from a single measurement of dialyzed urea. ASAIO Journal. 1995;**41**:M804-M809. DOI: 10.1097/00002480-199507000-00126

[70] Vanholder R, Argilés A, Jankowski J. European uraemic toxin work group (EUTox). A history of uraemic toxicity and of the European uraemic toxin work group (EUTox). Clinical Kidney Journal. 2021;**14**:1514-1523. DOI: 10.1093/ckj/sfab011

[71] Fridolin I, Lindberg LG. On-line monitoring of solutes in dialysate using wavelength-dependent absorption of ultraviolet radiation. Medical & Biological Engineering & Computing. 2003;**41**: 263-270. DOI: 10.1007/BF02348430

[72] Vanholder R, Argilés A, Baurmeister U, Brunet P, Clark W, Cohen G, et al. Uremic toxicity: Present state of the art. The International Journal of Artificial Organs. 2001;**24**:695-725

[73] Clark WR, Dehghani NL, Narsimhan V, Ronco C. Uremic toxins and their relation to dialysis efficacy. Blood Purification. 2019;**48**:299-314. DOI: 10.1159/000502331

[74] Rosner MH, Reis T, Husain-Syed F, Vanholder R, Hutchison C, Stenvinkel P, et al. Classification of uremic toxins and their role in kidney failure. Clinical Journal of the American Society of Nephrology. 2021;**16**:1918-1928. DOI: 10.2215/CJN.02660221

[75] Castillo-Rodríguez E, Pizarro-Sánchez S, Sanz AB, Ramos AM, Sanchez-Niño MD, Martin-Cleary C, et al. Inflammatory cytokines as uremic toxins. Toxins (Basel). 2017;**9**:114. DOI: 10.3390/toxins9040114

[76] Graboski AL, Redinbo MR. Gut-derived protein-bound uremic toxins. Toxins (Basel). 2020;**12**:590. DOI: 10.3390/toxins12090590

[77] Perego AF. Adsorption techniques: Dialysis sorbents and membranes. Blood Purification. 2013;**35**(Suppl. 2):48-51. DOI: 10.1159/000350848

[78] Vanholder R, Pletinck A, Schepers E, Glorieux G. Biochemical and clinical impact of organic uremic retention solutes: A comprehensive update. Toxins (Basel). 2018;**10**:33. DOI: 10.3390/toxins10010033

[79] Jerotskaja J, Uhlin F, Lauri K, Tanner R, Luman M, Fridolin I. A multicentre study of an enhanced optical method for measuring concentration of uric acid removed during dialysis. In: Annual International Conference of the IEEE Engineering in Medicine and Biology Society. Vol. 2009. New York City: IEEE; 2009. pp. 1477-1480. DOI: 10.1109/IEMBS.2009.5332433. PMID: 19963503

[80] Jerotskaja J, Uhlin F, Fridolin I, Lauri K, Luman M, Fernström A. Optical online monitoring of uric acid removal during dialysis. Blood Purification. 2010; **29**:69-74. DOI: 10.1159/000264269

[81] Holmar J, Fridolin I, Uhlin F, Lauri K, Luman M. Optical method for cardiovascular risk marker uric acid removal assessment during dialysis. The Scientific World Journal. 2012;**2012**: 506486. DOI: 10.1100/2012/506486

[82] Tomson R, Fridolin I, Uhlin F, Holmar J, Lauri K, Luman M. Optical measurement of creatinine in spent dialysate. Clinical Nephrology. 2013;**79**: 107-117. DOI: 10.5414/CN107338

[83] Uhlin F, Fridolin I. Optical monitoring of dialysis dose. In: Azar A, editor. Modeling and Control of Dialysis Systems. Studies in Computational Intelligence. Berlin: Springer; 2013. pp. 867-928. DOI: 10.1007/978-3-642-27558-6_3

[84] Enberg P, Fridolin I, Holmar J, Fernström A, Uhlin F. Utilization of UV absorbance for estimation of phosphate elimination during hemodiafiltration. Nephron. Clinical Practice. 2012;**121**:c1-c9. DOI: 10.1159/000341598

[85] Holmar J, Uhlin F, Fernström A, Luman M, Jankowski J, Fridolin I. An optical method for serum calcium and phosphorus level assessment during

hemodialysis. Toxins (Basel). 2015;7: 719-727. DOI: 10.3390/toxins7030719

[86] Uhlin F, Holmar J, Yngman-Uhlin P, Fernström A, Fridolin I. Optical estimation of beta 2 microglobulin during hemodiafiltration – does it work? Blood Purification. 2015;**40**:113-119. DOI: 10.1159/000381797

[87] Holmar J, Arund J, Uhlin F, Tanner R, Fridolin I. Beta2-microglobulin measurements in the spent dialysate using fluorescence spectra. In: 5th European Conference of the International Federation for Medical and Biological Engineering; 14–18 September 2011; Budapest. Hungary. Berlin: Springer; 2011. pp. 1035-1038

[88] Miyata T, Oda O, Inagi R, Iida Y, Araki N, Yamada N, et al. beta 2-Microglobulin modified with advanced glycation end products is a major component of hemodialysis-associated amyloidosis. The Journal of Clinical Investigation. 1993;**92**:1243-1252. DOI: 10.1172/JCI116696

[89] Kalle S, Kressa H, Tanner R, Holmar J, Fridolin I. Fluorescence of beta-2-microglobulin in the spent dialysate. In: Mindedal H, Persson M, editors. 16th Nordic-Baltic Conference on Biomedical Engineering. IFMBE Proceedings. Vol. 48. Göteborg. Cham: Springer; 2015. pp. 59-62. DOI: 10.1007/978-3-319-12967-9_16

[90] Paats J, Adoberg A, Arund J, Fridolin I, Lauri K, Leis L, et al. Optical method and biochemical source for the assessment of the middle-molecule uremic toxin β2-microglobulin in spent dialysate. Toxins (Basel). 2021;**13**:255. DOI: 10.3390/toxins13040255

[91] Holmar J, Uhlin F, Ferenets R, Lauri K, Tanner R, Arund J, et al. Estimation of removed uremic toxin indoxyl sulphate during hemodialysis by using optical data of the spent dialysate. In: 2013 35th Annual International Conference of the IEEE Engineering in Medicine and Biology Society (EMBC). New York City: IEEE; 2013. pp. 6707-6710. DOI: 10.1109/EMBC.2013.6611095

[92] Arund J, Luman M, Uhlin F, Tanner R, Fridolin I. Is fluorescence valid to monitor removal of protein bound uremic solutes in dialysis? PLoS One. 2016;**11**:e0156541. DOI: 10.1371/journal.pone.0156541

[93] Barnett AL, Veening H. Liquid-chromatographic study of fluorescent compounds in hemodialysate solutions. Clinical Chemistry. 1985;**31**:127-130

[94] Swan JS, Kragten EY, Veening H. Liquid-chromatographic study of fluorescent materials in uremic fluids. Clinical Chemistry. 1983;**29**:1082-1084

[95] Pilt K, Arund J, Adoberg A, Leis L, Luman M, Fridolin I. Intradialytic on-line multicomponent reduction ratio monitoring in spent dialysate by a novel miniaturized optical sensor. In: 46th ESAO Congress; 3–7 September 2019. Hannover. Germany: SAGE Publications Ltd STM; 2019;**42**(8):386-474. DOI: 10.1177/0391398819860985

[96] Fridolin I. A concept for smart real-time monitoring of intermittent renal replacement therapy. In: 46th ESAO Congress; 3–7 September 2019. Hannover. The International Journal of Artificial Organs. Germany: SAGE Publications Ltd STM; 2019;**42**(8):386-474. DOI: 10.1177/0391398819860985

[97] Adoberg A, Paats J, Arund J, Leis L, Pilt K, Fridolin I, et al. Intradialytic on-line multicomponent total removed solute monitoring in spent dialysate by a novel miniaturized optical sensor. In:

57th ERA-EDTA Congress, Fully Virtual, Nephrology Dialysis Transplantation, Volume 35, Issue Supplement_3. Oxford: Oxford Academic; 2020. DOI: 10.1093/ndt/gfaa141.TO015

[98] Leis L, Adoberg A, Paats J, Arund J, Pilt K, Luman M, et al. Intradialytic online multicomponent total removed solute monitoring in spent dialysate by a novel miniaturized optical sensor. In: Kidney Week. Journal of American Society of Nephrology. Alphen aan den Rijn, The Netherlands: Wolters Kluwer; 19-25 October 2020. pp. 370-371

[99] Lin K-Y, Liang C-S, Hsu C-C, Lin S-L, Chen Y-T, Huang F-S, et al. Optoelectronic online monitoring system for hemodialysis and its data analysis. Sensors and Actuators B: Chemical. 2022; **364**:131859. ISSN 0925-4005. DOI: 10.1016/j.snb.2022.131859

[100] Arund J, Tanner R, Uhlin F, Fridolin I. Do only small uremic toxins, chromophores, contribute to the online dialysis dose monitoring by UV absorbance? Toxins (Basel). 2012;**4**: 849-861. DOI: 10.3390/toxins4100849

[101] Adoberg A, Paats J, Arund J, Dhondt A, Fridolin I, Glorieux G, et al. Treatment with paracetamol can interfere with the intradialytic optical estimation in spent dialysate of uric acid but not of indoxyl sulfate. Toxins (Basel). 2022;**14**:610. DOI: 10.3390/toxins14090610

[102] Kalle S, Tanner R, Luman M, Fridolin I. Free pentosidine assessment based on fluorescence measurements in spent dialysate. Blood Purification. 2019; **47**:85-93. DOI: 10.1159/000493522

[103] Paats J, Adoberg A, Arund J, Dhondt A, Fernström A, Fridolin I, et al. Serum levels and removal by hemodialysis and hemodiafiltration of tryptophan-derived uremic toxins in ESKD patients. International Journal of Molecular Sciences. 2020;**21**:1522. DOI: 10.3390/ijms21041522

[104] Adoberg A, Leis L, Uhlin F, Arund J, Segelmark M, Fernström A, et al. Combined displacer-enhanced removal of protein-bound uremic toxins estimated in spent dialysate. In: International Society of Nephrology, ISN World Congress of Nephrology; 12–15 April 2019. In: Kidney International Reports. Melbourne. Australia: International Society of Nephrology; 2019. pp. S340-S341. Available from: https://cm.theisn.org/cmPortal/Searchable/WCN2019/config/normal#!abstractde

[105] Arund J, Adoberg A, Leis L, Luman M, Uhlin F, Segelmark M, et al. Optical on-line monitoring of a displacer-chromophore administration during a dialysis treatment. In: International Society of Nephrology, ISN World Congress of Nephrology; 12–15 April 2019. In: Kidney International Reports. Melbourne. Australia: International Society of Nephrology; 2019. pp. S340-S341. Available from: https://cm.theisn.org/cmPortal/Searchable/WCN2019/config/normal#!abstractde

Chapter 4

Innovations in Hemodialysis Access

Nidharshan S. Anandasivam and Tessa K. Novick

Abstract

The established types of vascular access for hemodialysis are central venous catheters (CVCs), arteriovenous fistulas (AVFs), and arteriovenous grafts (AVGs). Innovations in CVC tip and coating design may improve patency and blood flow rates. AVFs are preferred over CVCs as they are less prone to clotting and infection, while providing reliable and adequate blood flow rates. However, AVF creation requires a surgical procedure with associated risks. Because of a paucity of surgeons available to create high-quality dialysis access, newer access creation techniques have been developed, including a percutaneous endovascular method that has the potential to revolutionize dialysis access. Innovations in AVGs include drug-eluting devices that may reduce neointimal hyperplasia and bioengineered blood vessels. To bypass vessel stenoses, a hybrid AVG/CVC device has been developed. Although many of these innovations have yet to become mainstream, they promise to improve dialysis access in the future.

Keywords: hemodialysis access, arteriovenous fistula, percutaneous arteriovenous fistula, central venous catheter, arteriovenous grafts (AVGs)

1. Introduction

Hemodialysis is the most common modality of dialysis worldwide for patients with end-stage kidney disease (ESKD). In the US, approximately 786,000 patients have ESKD, and 71% of these patients are on dialysis, while 29% have received a kidney transplant [1]. Optimal vascular access is essential for hemodialysis to achieve adequate blood flow rates and maintain patency, while minimizing the risk of complications such as infection and thrombosis.

The most common options for vascular access for hemodialysis are central venous catheters (CVCs), arteriovenous fistulas (AVFs), and arteriovenous grafts (AVGs). AVFs are generally preferred over CVCs due to lower complications overall, reliable blood flow rates, and reduced need for corrective procedures. In those with tunneled CVCs, the likelihood of catheter-related bacteremia is 35% at 3 months and 48% at 6 months [2]. Patients with CVCs experience 4.6 catheter-related bacteremia episodes/1000 catheter-days [2]. Furthermore, up to 40% of catheter-related bloodstream infections lead to further complications such as osteomyelitis and endocarditis [3]. In a study of 865 dialysis patients, catheter dysfunction occurred at a rate of 10.58 episodes/1000 catheter-days and affected 56.65% of patients [4]. Other known risks of CVCs include catheter lumen thrombosis and central venous stenosis [2]. Compared to AVFs, CVCs have shown to have higher infection-related deaths

IntechOpen

(RR = 2.30, $p < 0.05$), higher cardiac-related deaths (RR = 1.47, $p < 0.05$), and higher overall mortality risk (RR = 1.54, $p < 0.05$) [5]. Despite the plethora of evidence of AVFs demonstrating better outcomes compared to CVCs, certain vulnerable populations, like those receiving emergency-only hemodialysis (EOHD), are less likely to start their first dialysis with an AVF compared to standard hemodialysis patients [6]. This suggests that there are barriers to receiving timely optimal vascular access, and many would benefit from innovations in hemodialysis access.

The possibility of converting AVF creation from a mainstream surgical procedure to a mainstream interventional procedure holds promise for improving access for patients with CVCs in need of AVFs. This chapter will examine innovations in hemodialysis access as it pertains to CVCs, AVFs, and AVGs.

2. Central venous catheters

Central venous catheters are used widely for hemodialysis access. Non-tunneled catheters are used for emergent dialysis access and are common in the intensive care setting. Tunneled catheters are placed for hemodialysis access in urgent, but non-emergent, cases in hospitalized patients. Tunneled CVCs can be functional for over a year, but dysfunction and complications are not uncommon. Although CVCs have been associated with worse outcomes compared to AVFs and AVGs, they are still pervasive because they can be placed easily and utilized immediately. Furthermore, accessing CVCs avoids the needlesticks required for AVFs and AVGs. Despite this, it is generally recommended to use CVCs only as a bridge to AVFs because of the common complications of CVCs, or when individuals have limited life expectancy and the risks of AVF or AVG creation do not outweigh benefits. CVCs can be either non-tunneled (for emergent short-term use) or tunneled through subcutaneous tissue (for longer-term use on the order of months), and both are associated with higher morbidity and mortality compared to AVFs. Over the last several years, the design of CVCs has improved to maximize blood flow rate, minimize endothelial injury, improve catheter function and biocompatibility, and minimize infections [7].

Catheter tip design has evolved from step tip to split tip to symmetric tip, with the goal of preventing thrombosis and recirculation of blood (**Figure 1**) [8]. The difference lies in the end of the catheter. The step tip catheter has its two ends offset by a distance, while the split tip catheter has a Y-shaped end with the two tips diverging. The symmetric tip catheter as the two ends of the catheter adjacent and mirroring each other. One study of 302 patients examined split tip and symmetric tip designs and found no difference in mean primary assisted patency [9]. One study found lower recirculation rates with the symmetric tip (0% for symmetric tip vs. 22.3–39.2% for split tip vs. 8.7–16.3% for step tip) [10]. A study comparing split tip and step tip catheters found that the step tip catheter delivered higher blood flow rates (433 mL/min vs. 414 mL/min), but both types were able to deliver blood flow rates that were well above that recommended by the Dialysis Outcomes Quality Initiative [11]. Overall, there have been mixed results, and it is inconclusive which design is optimal.

In theory, catheter coatings can be utilized externally and internally to prevent biofilm formation and activation of the coagulation cascade, which would prevent infection and thrombosis. Catheters can be coated with heparin to prevent thrombosis and antibiotics to prevent infection. However, a systematic review examining coatings have failed to show significant benefit [12].

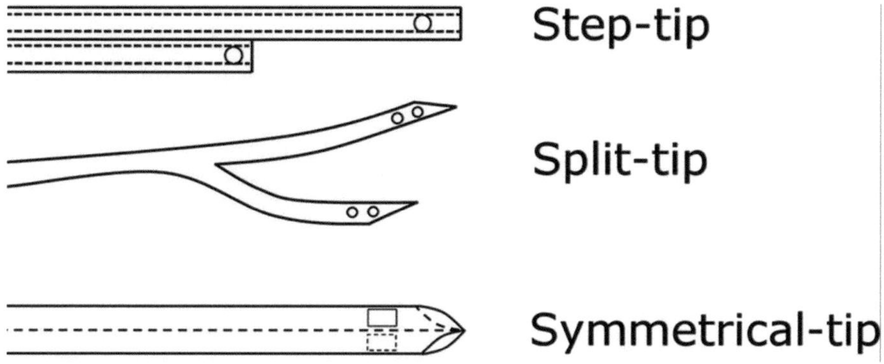

Figure 1.
Catheter designs. This illustrates three common types of catheter designs for hemodialysis access. The goal of the evolution from step tip to split tip to symmetric tip was to prevent thrombosis and blood recirculation. Although a few studies have demonstrated certain advantages for each, it is inconclusive which design is optimal overall. Reprinted from: [8] Copyright 2019, with permission from Elsevier. This is an Open Access article distributed under the terms of the Creative Commons Attribution License (https://creativecommons.org/licenses/by/4.0/).

Although early catheters were made of silicone, newer polyurethane/polycarbonate polymers are used to increase luminal diameter (thin walls) while maintaining strength, flexibility, and rigidity to prevent luminal collapse at high negative pressures [13]. Large randomized controlled studies comparing catheter materials are lacking.

Catheter lock solutions have been used for the purposes of antisepsis (antimicrobials) and anticoagulation (heparin or citrate). There is weak positive evidence that antibacterial lock solutions decrease the incidence of catheter-related bloodstream infection [14]. To date, there has not been an ideal catheter lock solution that has reliably prevented infection or catheter dysfunction. It is controversial whether we should use antibiotic locks to treat catheter-related blood stream infections, as the evidence supporting this is minimal, and only includes small observational studies [15].

3. Arteriovenous fistulas

In 1966, Brescia et. al. created a connection between an artery and a vein and allowed it to mature giving rise to the AVF [16]. This was groundbreaking in delivering optimal blood flow for hemodialysis. Initial side-to-side anastomoses had issues with hand edema, so it was further refined to end-to-end anastomoses to prevent this. Even today, AVFs have lower infection rates and better patency than CVCs, as they remain the ideal option for dialysis access.

In the last decade, endovascular techniques have been devised to create AVFs, revolutionizing dialysis access creation with the power to improve patient access to high-quality AVFs. Two novel devices for endovascular interventions have been approved by the US Food and Drug Administration.

The first device, the everlinQ endoAVF system (TVA Medical, Austin, TX), was studied in the Novel Endovascular Access Trial (**Figure 2**) [17, 18]. This uses radiofrequency energy and catheter technology to create an AVF. Specifically in this procedure, the brachial vein is penetrated with a needle and guidewire, which is then passed into the ulnar vein. Separately, the brachial artery is punctured in an antegrade direction, and a guidewire is advanced to the ulnar artery. A venous magnetic catheter is introduced into the ulnar vein, while an arterial magnetic catheter is introduced

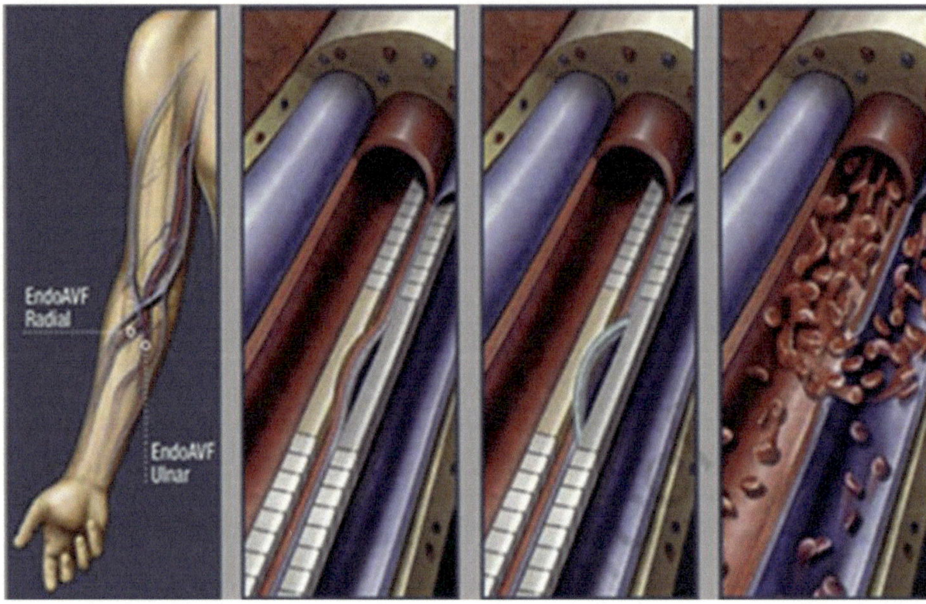

Figure 2.
EverlinQ EndoAVF system. This system allows for an endovascular approach to creation of an arteriovenous fistula (AVF). A venous magnetic catheter is introduced into the vein, while an arterial magnetic catheter is introduced into the artery. An anastomosis between the vein and artery is created as the magnetic catheters are aligned, allowing for activation of a radiofrequency electrode and creation of an AVF. Reprinted from: [17]. Copyright 2022, with permission from Elsevier. This is an Open Access article distributed under the terms of the Creative Commons Attribution License (https://creativecommons.org/licenses/by/4.0/).

into the ulnar artery. An anastomosis is created between the ulnar artery and vein as the magnetic catheters are aligned, allowing for activation of a radiofrequency electrode. In the trial examining 59 AVFs created using this technique, the primary and cumulative patency at 12 months were 69 and 84%, respectively. Mean time for fistula maturation was 111 days [18].

The second device used to create an AVF is the thermal resistance anastomosis device (TRAD) [19]. This uses thermal resistance energy to create an anastomosis between a vein and artery. In this procedure, a needle cannulates the vein (usually brachial or cubital) in a retrograde fashion using ultrasound, and then punctures into the proximal radial artery, allowing a guidewire to follow. Next, the TRAD advances into the vein-artery junction and creates a durable anastomosis. Angioplasty is done afterwards to augment flow into this anastomosis. In a study examining 107 percutaneous AVFs created using this Ellipsys Vascular Access System (Avenu Medical, San Juan Capistrano, CA), cumulative patency at 90, 180, and 360 days was 91.6, 89.3, and 86.7%, respectively [19].

These early results demonstrate that AVFs can be created through endovascular intervention, with reliable function afterwards. This can be accomplished by interventionalists without general anesthesia. If this were to become mainstream, patients needing dialysis access creation would have many more options rather than the necessity of waiting to see a vascular surgeon for AVF creation. Access to dialysis creation would be revolutionized.

Far infrared therapy has been studied for its effects in improving maturation and patency of newly created AVFs [20]. These are electromagnetic waves that may improve cutaneous blood flow. Many theorized mechanisms have been postulated for how it may improve AVF function, including thermal effects, inflammation suppression, and decreased oxidative injury. In a randomized controlled study of 122 patients, 62 patients received 40 minutes of far infrared therapy 3 times weekly for a year. The intervention group had a higher blood flow rate, a lower occurrence of AVF malfunction (12% vs. 29%, p = 0.02), and more cumulative unassisted patency (87% vs. 70%, p = 0.01) within 12 months [20].

Neointimal hyperplasia presents a challenge to the patency of vascular access. Because of this, it is a therapeutic target. Vonapanitase (recombinant human elastase) has been studied in a randomized controlled trial to determine if it improved primary and secondary patency [21]. It is known to disrupt elastin and other peptides that may attract cell proliferation, and has potential benefit in improving AVF patency. When applied during radiocephalic AVF creation, vonapanitase reduced primary (HR = 0.37, p = 0.02) and secondary (HR = 0.24, p = 0.046) patency loss. It also was associated with fewer procedures to restore or maintain fistula patency. However, there was no significant difference in risk of primary patency loss with vonapanitase overall in this study. Further research is essential to evaluate the efficacy of vonapanitase in improving dialysis access patency.

4. Arteriovenous grafts

AVGs constitute about 12–13% of vascular accesses in Europe, Japan, Australia, and New Zealand, compared to 25% in the United States [22]. Although AVFs are much more common than AVGs, both are preferred over CVCs. AVGs may be preferable over AVFs when a patient has unsuitable veins for AVF or AVF maturation issues. A study examining mortality in maintenance hemodialysis patients showed that transitioning from a CVC to an AVG of AVF was associated with reduced mortality (hazard ratio [HR] = 0.69), and transitioning from AVG or AVF to a CVC was associated with higher mortality (HR = 2.12) [23].

In the past, AVG advances have focused on reducing vein stenosis and graft clotting, as well as altering flow dynamics. Recent advances in AVGs include early cannulation AVGs (eAVGs), anti-neointimal hyperplasia AVG therapy, hybrid AVGs, and bioengineered vessels as AVGs.

The eAVG is a graft that can be cannulated within 72 hours of placement for dialysis. It is designed to with materials to prevent back wall puncture, and with self-sealing properties to allow for immediate access [24]. One 2015 systematic review showed that eAVGs had similar complication and patency rates to standard AVGs made of expanded polytetrafluoroethylene (ePTFE) [25].

Another advance in AVG technology relies on surface modification. Heparin coatings have been created to lower the risk of thrombosis, although the evidence on whether it reduces thrombosis is controversial [26]. Other efforts have been made to make grafts more biocompatible through strategies such as outer wall modification using electrospinning, nanotopography, or lithography. To combat neointimal hyperplasia, which causes graft failure, sirolimus-eluting devices and paclitaxel coatings have been designed. Although a few studies have demonstrated successful use of these anti-proliferative agents, large comparative trials are lacking [27, 28].

Hybrid AVG systems have allowed navigation through central vein stenosis. The Hemodialysis Reliable Outflow device (HeRO, Merit Medical Systems, South Jordan, UT), uses a combination of a tunneled CVC and AVG to provide hemodialysis access while bypassing a venous stenosis or occlusion (**Figure 3**) [29]. Although expensive,

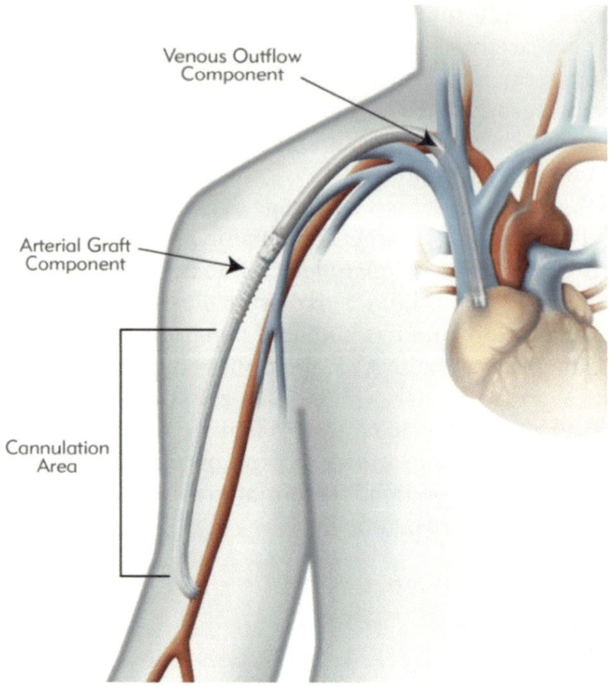

Figure 3.
Hemodialysis reliable outflow (HeRO) Graft. This illustrates the HeRO Graft, which utilizes an expanded polytetrafluoroethylene (ePTFE) component to bypass venous stenoses and occlusions. The graft is anastomosed to an artery on one end and is inserted into a central vein on the other end, bypassing the stenosis/occlusion in between. Reprinted from: HeRO Graft [Internet]. Merit Medical; 2022. Available from: https://www.merit.com/peripheral-intervention/access/renal-therapies-accessories/merit-hero-graft/. Copyright 2022, from Merit Medical. © Merit Medical, Reprinted by Permission.

this device may save cost due to lower complications compared to a tunneled CVC alone [30].

Over the last few decades, tissue bioengineered vessels have been created to replace prosthetic grafts. Blood vessels may be chemically treated to decrease immunogenicity. Human vascular cells may be grown on biodegradable scaffolds. One study in the US and Poland investigating human acellular vessels found that after a year, primary patency was 28% and secondary patency was 89% [31]. Overall, these bioengineered vessels have demonstrated better patency than standard AVGs in a few studies, but evidence of clinical benefit over standard AVGs is lacking.

5. Conclusion

Innovations in CVCs, AVFs, and AVGs over the last several decades have revolutionized care for patients needing long-term dialysis. The main challenges in assuring adequate hemodialysis access include timing and logistics of obtaining an AVF, preventing access stenosis and thrombosis, and preventing infection. The abovementioned innovations are cornerstones in improving quality of care in patients undergoing long-term hemodialysis. Overall, more research into the efficacy of these innovations, as well as larger comparative trials, are needed to gain the public's trust and bring these innovations into the mainstream. However, the wealth of literature

DOI: http://dx.doi.org/10.5772/intechopen.110467

on these hemodialysis access improvements suggests that the future will not only see incremental improvements in CVCs and AVGs, but also stark changes to the way hemodialysis access is achieved with inventions like the endoAVF and HeRO. Obtaining and sustaining optimal durable vascular access for hemodialysis is a complex and challenging task, but these innovations promise to build on our current quality of hemodialysis access.

Author details

Nidharshan S. Anandasivam* and Tessa K. Novick
Department of Internal Medicine, Dell Medical School at the University of Texas at Austin, Austin, TX, United States

*Address all correspondence to: nidharshan17@gmail.com

References

[1] Johansen KL, Chertow GM, Foley RN, Gilbertson DT, Herzog CA, Ishani A, et al. US renal data system 2020 annual data report: Epidemiology of kidney disease in the United States. American Journal of Kidney Diseases. 2021;**77** (4 Suppl. 1):A7-A8

[2] Lee T, Barker J, Allon M. Tunneled catheters in hemodialysis patients: Reasons and subsequent outcomes. American Journal of Kidney Disease. 2005;**46**(3):501-508

[3] Fisher M, Golestaneh L, Allon M, Abreo K, Mokrzycki MH. Prevention of bloodstream infections in patients undergoing hemodialysis. Clinical Journal of the American Society of Nephrology. 2020;**15**(1):132-151

[4] Wang K, Wang P, Liang X, Lu X, Liu Z. Epidemiology of haemodialysis catheter complications: A survey of 865 dialysis patients from 14 haemodialysis centres in Henan province in China. BMJ Open. 2015;**5**(11):e007136

[5] Dhingra RK, Young EW, Hulbert-Shearon TE, Leavey SF, Port FK. Type of vascular access and mortality in U.S. hemodialysis patients. Kidney International. 2001;**60**(4):1443-1451

[6] Cervantes L, Tuot D, Raghavan R, Linas S, Zoucha J, Sweeney L, et al. Association of emergency-only vs standard hemodialysis with mortality and health care use among undocumented immigrants with end-stage renal disease. JAMA Internal Medicine. 2018;**178**(2):188-195

[7] Agarwal AK, Haddad NJ, Vachharajani TJ, Asif A. Innovations in vascular access for hemodialysis. Kidney International. 2019;**95**(5):1053-1063

[8] Ling XC, Lu HP, Loh EW, Lin YK, Li YS, Lin CH, et al. A systematic review and meta-analysis of the comparison of performance among step-tip, split-tip, and symmetrical-tip hemodialysis catheters. Journal of Vascular Surgery. 2019;**69**(4):1282-1292. DOI: 10.1016/j.jvs.2018.09.029

[9] Van Der Meersch H, De Bacquer D, Vandecasteele SJ, Van den Bergh B, Vermeiren P, De Letter J, et al. Hemodialysis catheter design and catheter performance: A randomized controlled trial. American Journal of Kidney Disease. 2014;**64**(6):902-908

[10] Vesely TM, Ravenscroft A. Hemodialysis catheter tip design: Observations on fluid flow and recirculation. The Journal of Vascular Access. 2016;**17**(1):29-39

[11] Trerotola SO, Kraus M, Shah H, Namyslowski J, Johnson MS, Stecker MS, et al. Randomized comparison of split tip versus step tip high-flow hemodialysis catheters. Kidney International. 2002;**62**(1):282-289

[12] Gilbert RE, Harden M. Effectiveness of impregnated central venous catheters for catheter related blood stream infection: A systematic review. Current Opinion in Infectious Diseases. 2008;**21**(3):235-245

[13] Ash SR. The evolution and function of central venous catheters for dialysis. Seminars in Dialysis. 2001;**14**(6):416-424

[14] Arechabala MC, Catoni MI, Claro JC, Rojas NP, Rubio ME, Calvo MA, et al. Antimicrobial lock solutions for preventing catheter-related infections in haemodialysis. Cochrane Database of Systematic Reviews. 2018;**4**(4):CD010597

[15] Labriola L. Antibiotic locks for the treatment of catheter-related blood stream infection: Still more hope than data. Seminars in Dialysis. 2019;**32**(5):402-405

[16] Brescia MJ, Cimino JE, Appel K, Hurwich BJ. Chronic hemodialysis using venipuncture and a surgically created arteriovenous fistula. The New England Journal of Medicine. 1966;**275**(20):1089-1092

[17] Berland T, Clement J, Inston N, Kreienberg P, Ouriel K. Percutaneous arteriovenous fistula creation with the 4F WavelinQ EndoAVF System. Journal of Vascular Surgery. 2022;**75**(3):1038-1046.e3

[18] Lok CE, Rajan DK, Clement J, Kiaii M, Sidhu R, Thomson K, et al. Endovascular proximal forearm arteriovenous fistula for hemodialysis access: Results of the prospective, multicenter novel endovascular access trial (NEAT). American Journal of Kidney Disease. 2017;**70**(4):486-497

[19] Hull JE, Jennings WC, Cooper RI, Waheed U, Schaefer ME, Narayan R. The Pivotal Multicenter Trial of Ultrasound-Guided Percutaneous Arteriovenous Fistula Creation for Hemodialysis Access. Journal of Vascular and Interventional Radiology. 2018;**29**(2):149-158.e5

[20] Lin CC, Yang WC, Chen MC, Liu WS, Yang CY, Lee PC. Effect of far infrared therapy on arteriovenous fistula maturation: An open-label randomized controlled trial. American Journal of Kidney Disease. 2013;**62**(2):304-311

[21] Peden EK, O'Connor TP, Browne BJ, Dixon BS, Schanzer AS, Jensik SC, et al. Arteriovenous fistula patency in the 3 years following vonapanitase and placebo treatment. Journal of Vascular Surgery. 2017;**65**(4):1113-1120

[22] Pisoni RL, Zepel L, Fluck R, Lok CE, Kawanishi H, Süleymanlar G, et al. International differences in the location and use of arteriovenous accesses created for hemodialysis: Results from the dialysis outcomes and practice patterns study (DOPPS). American Journal of Kidney Diseases. 2018;**71**(4):469-478

[23] Lacson EJ, Wang W, Lazarus JM, Hakim RM. Change in vascular access and mortality in maintenance hemodialysis patients. American Journal of Kidney Diseases. 2009;**54**(5):912-921

[24] Gage SM, Lawson M, Nichols C, Sycks D, Manson RJ, Knight JA. An immediate access dialysis graft designed to prevent needle-related complications: Results from the initial pre-clinical studies. The Journal of Vascular Access. 2020;**21**(3):328-335

[25] Al Shakarchi J, Houston G, Inston N. Early cannulation grafts for haemodialysis: A systematic review. The Journal of Vascular Access. 2015;**16**(6):493-497

[26] Shemesh D, Goldin I, Hijazi J, Zaghal I, Berelowitz D, Verstandig A, et al. A prospective randomized study of heparin-bonded graft (Propaten) versus standard graft in prosthetic arteriovenous access. Journal of Vascular Surgery. 2015;**62**(1):115-122

[27] Paulson WD, Kipshidze N, Kipiani K, Beridze N, DeVita MV, Shenoy S, et al. Safety and efficacy of local periadventitial delivery of sirolimus for improving hemodialysis graft patency: First human experience with a sirolimus-eluting collagen membrane (Coll-R). Nephrology Dialysis Transplantation. 2012;**27**(3):1219-1224

[28] Baek I, Bai CZ, Hwang J, Nam HY, Park JS, Kim DJ. Paclitaxel coating of the luminal surface of hemodialysis grafts

with effective suppression of neointimal hyperplasia. Journal of Vascular Surgery. 2012;**55**(3):806-814.e1

[29] HeRO Graft [Internet]. Merit Medical. Available from: https://www.merit.com/peripheral-intervention/access/renal-therapies-accessories/merit-hero-graft/

[30] Al Shakarchi J, Inston N, Jones RG, Maclaine G, Hollinworth D. Cost analysis of the Hemodialysis Reliable Outflow (HeRO) Graft compared to the tunneled dialysis catheter. Journal of Vascular Surgery. 2016;**63**(4):1026-1033

[31] Lawson JH, Glickman MH, Ilzecki M, Jakimowicz T, Jaroszynski A, Peden EK, et al. Bioengineered human acellular vessels for dialysis access in patients with end-stage renal disease: Two phase 2 single-arm trials. Lancet. 2016;**387**(10032):2026-2034

Chapter 5

Acute Complication during Hemodialysis

Saurav Singh Hamal and Pratima Khadka

Abstract

Haemodialysis was first done successfully in humans, in 1945, and since then a lot of technological advancements have been made, there are still common acute complications that are encountered by physicians during their routine practice. The common complications include intradialytic hypotension, hypertension, arrhythmias, muscle cramps, sudden cardiac death, headache, etc., occurring in about 10–70% of patients undergoing haemodialysis. The mechanism of these complications is multifactorial and treatment of these complications is important to prevent mortality of the patients. Prevention is important including multiple disciplinary approaches. Here we discuss some of the common complications that occur in routine haemodialysis sessions.

Keywords: haemodialysis, blood flow rate, ultrafiltration, dialysate, heparin

1. Introduction

Haemodialysis was first done successfully in humans, in 1945, and since then a lot of technological advancements have been made [1].

There are still common acute complications that are encountered by physicians during their routine practice. The common complications include intradialytic hypotension and hypertension, muscle cramps, clotting of the circuit and dialyzer reactions. Some are severe and lead to increase mortality of the patients hence they need to be identified and treated early, some are mild, which again need early identification and management to avoid cumbersome tests and intervention. These are discussed briefly below, under systematic headings.

2. Acute complications during haemodialysis

We will discuss some of the common acute complications that occur during routine haemodialysis sessions and are categorized as below:

2.1 Cardiovascular complications

The common cardiovascular complication that may occur during haemodialysis include:

2.1.1 Intradialytic hypotension (IDH)

IDH is defined as, decrease in systolic blood pressure by ≥20 mmHg or a decrease in MAP of ≥10 mmHg associated with symptoms of dizziness, restlessness or need for intervention by a supporting staff. It occurs in about 10–40% of dialysis treatment, the discrepancy in prevalence is not known exactly but may be due to use of various definition of IDH (**Table 1**) [1, 2].

Pathogenesis of IDH is complex and includes:

1. Excessive ultrafiltration.
2. Reduce plasma filling.
3. Cardiac disease.
4. Dialyzer reaction.
5. Haemolysis.

Leading to reduced effective circulating volume and subsequently intradialytic hypotension.

Clinical features include; abdominal discomfort, nausea and vomiting, muscle cramp, dizziness and anxiety.

IDH is associated with several notable clinical consequences, the most common are cardiovascular events and mortality.

It is associated with myocardial stunning, a reversible phenomenon that occurs due to repetitive ischemia with each episode of IDH and may initiate myocardial fibrosis and irreversible systolic dysfunction. Similarly reduced cerebral perfusion with each episode of IDH is associated with an increased risk of new-onset dementia. IDH also accelerates the loss of residual renal function with repeated episodes of hypotension, and less commonly IDH is also associated with vascular access thrombosis and mesenteric and liver ischemia.

Management strategy includes:

Several approaches have been suggested to treat IDH which include:

1. Immediate treatment:
    - Placing the patient in Trendelenburg position.
    - I.V bolus of 0.9% normal saline >100 ml, and slowing the UF to allow time for plasma refill and restoration of B.P.
    - Observing for hemodynamic status and subsequently managing patient further.
2. Prevention
    - Adjusting dialysis prescription:
        a. A cool dialysate below core body temperature induces vasoconstriction and activates sympathetic nervous system decreasing the risk of IDH.

b. Adjusting UF rate to ≤10 ml/kg/hr, as UF rate above >10 ml/kg/hr has been associated with an increased risk of a cardiovascular event and all-cause mortality.

c. Adjusting dialysate sodium concentration has shown conflicting results, and hence no current recommendation can be given.

d. Technique like hemofiltration outcome on mortality is still controversial and cannot be recommended for now.

e. Use of drugs, midodrine an alpha 1 adrenergic receptor agonist, was associated with increased mortality and should not be used routinely.

f. Lowering antihypertensive drugs on dialysis days can be an option that needs to be compared in randomized trials.

g. Switching to PD is one of the alternatives to avoid intradialytic hypotension, as IDH is rarely seen in a patient undergoing PD.

2.1.2 Intradialytic hypertension

Intradialytic hypertension is a paradoxical rise in blood pressure that occurs during a haemodialysis procedure. it is another common complication that occurs in about 8–30% of dialysis sessions and is associated with high mortality [1, 3].

There are no accepted criteria, however, is commonly defined as a rise of systolic blood pressure >10 mmHg during HD, a rise of MAP > 15 mmHg during or immediately post-HD and/or any rise of blood pressure during HD.

	Decrease in SBP (mmHg)	Decrease in MAP (mmHg)	Symptoms or need for intervention
KDOQI clinical practice guidelines (2005)	≥20	≥10	Symptoms.
European Best practice (2007)	≥20	≥20	Symptoms and intervention.
UK renal association guidelines (2011)	Any	Any	Immediate intervention

Table 1.
Different definitions of intradialytic hypotension.

Etiopathogenesis of interdialytic hypertension includes:

Pathogenesis of intradialytic hypertension is unknown. However, it represents a state of volume overload, sympathetic overactivity, RAAS activation, endothelial dysfunction, increased level of endothelin 1, ESAs and sodium loading during dialysis.

Treatment includes:

During dialysis treatment should be done once SBP >180 mmHg during dialysis.

Interdialytic hypertension is best treated with drugs like clonidine or RAAS blockers like enalapril, other antihypertensive agents can be used as well.

Preventive measures include:

1. Optimization of dry weight.

2. Adjustment of antihypertensive agents:

There are several antihypertensive agents used in a patient under maintenance dialysis and the knowledge of dializability will help in adjusting the dose of drugs. The dialyzable drugs need to be repeated after a haemodialysis session (**Table 2**).

1. Adjustment of ESAs.

2. Consider low dialysate sodium about 136 mmol/l have shown to reduce incidence of intradialytic hypertension.

In a study performed in haemodialysis patients, dry weight reduction in hypertensive haemodialysis patients (DRIP) suggested that optimal control of BP in HD is via control of extracellular fluid volume and not the use of antihypertensive agents [4].

2.1.3 Arrhythmias

Intradialytic arrhythmias are common and are often multifactorial in origin, it represents a bad prognostic sign hence early identification and treatment are of paramount importance [5].

Bradycardia and asystole are more common followed by ventricular arrhythmias.

Antihypertensive agents	Dialysable	Not dialyzable
Calcium channel blocker		
Amlodipine		√
Verapamil		√
ARBs		
Losartan		√
Telmisartan		√
ACEi		
Enalapril	√	
Fosinopril		√
Beta-blocker		
Carvedilol		√
Metoprolol succinate	√	
Atenolol	√	
Bisoprolol		√
Others		
Clonidine		√
Prazosin		√

Table 2.
List of common antihypertensive drugs in haemodialysis patients.

Pathophysiology of intradialytic arrhythmias:

The pre-existing cardiac structural abnormality along with the acid-base disorder, electrolyte imbalance and dialysate component creates an arrhythmogenic milieu. And patients under maintenance dialysis are at increased risk of arrhythmias.

Clinical presentation can range from asymptomatic patients to patients presenting with palpitations, chest pain, dizziness, syncope and sudden cardiac death.

Management includes:

1. Immediate treatment: maintaining hemodynamic stability.

2. Preventive strategy includes:

- Complete cardiac evaluation and treating the type of arrhythmias with anti-arrhythmic drugs or devices.

- Adjusting dialysate content:

- A low calcium dialysate of <2.5 mEq/L have been associated with an increased risk of sudden cardiac death.

- A low potassium dialysate <2 mEq/L has been associated with an increased risk of sudden cardiac death.

- A high bicarbonate dialysate should be avoided, the optimum level is chosen empirically to correct metabolic acidosis.

2.1.4 Sudden death

Cardiac arrest is more common in elderly, diabetes, and patient using central venous catheters [5].

Aetiology is complex and related to pre-existing cardiac disease coupled with uremic milieu, that is inappropriate management of fluid volume and inadequate uremic toxins clearance [3, 4].

When sudden cardiac arrest occurs during dialysis, an immediate decision is to be made whether it is due to intrinsic cardiac disease or technical errors like air embolism, line disconnection, or sterilant in the dialyzer [5].

If no obvious cause is identified, blood should not be returned to patient.

Standard CPR should be performed.

2.2 Neuromuscular complication

2.2.1 Muscle cramps

Muscle cramps are a common cause of intradialytic discomfort and a frequent complication with an incidence of 5–20% in haemodialysis sessions [6].

It frequently involves the leg and leads to premature termination of haemodialysis.

Pathogenesis is unknown and largely attributed to dialysis-induced volume contraction and hypo-osmolality.

Management strategy includes increasing plasma osmolality by infusion of hypertonic saline (15 ml of 23.5%), or 50% dextrose in water (25–50 ml), or mannitol

25% (50 ml) [6, 7]. Evaluating for other causes of muscle cramps like thyroid disorder and electrolyte disturbances.

Prevention includes dietary counselling about excessive weight gain.

Beneficial effects of quinine sulphate (250–300 mg) or oxazepam (5 mg) given two hours prior to dialysis have been seen in some studies.

In some of the studies, vitamins E, L-carnitine, and enalapril have been used with some success [7].

2.2.2 Restless leg syndrome (RLS)

It was described in 1944 by K. A. Ekbom and is frequently seen in CKD patients particularly women with crawling leg sensation in leg and a compulsive need to move the limbs, usually leg. It affects 6.6–62% of patients on long-term dialysis [8].

Etiopathogenesis:

It can be familial in about 50% of patients, other risk factors include iron deficiency or iron transport into the CNS, which led to defects in iron homeostasis and downregulation of striatal dopamine receptors.

Management includes:

- Assess iron store and consider appropriate repletion.
- Asses other co-existing sleep disorders and assess drugs causing RLS.
- Non-pharmacologic treatment includes: avoid alcohol and caffeine.

Drugs: use of alpha2-delta calcium channel ligands such as gabapentin, pregabalin and dopamine agonist like pramipexole 0.125–0.5 mg at night are used, the mechanism of how they act is not known, and opioids have been used with some success.

Optimising dialysis with increased duration and frequency has been associated with a decreased incidence of RLS in FREEDOM study [9]. Middle molecules like alpha1 microglobulin have been linked to recurrence of restless leg syndrome in patient undergoing hemodialysis in small studies, however, more data are needed to reach into conclusion.

RLS improves in most of patients after kidney transplantation.

2.2.3 Seizures

It occurs in <10% of patients during dialysis and tends to be generalized. Focal seizure warrants evaluation for focal neurological cause [10].

Causes of seizure during haemodialysis include:

1. Drugs: erythropoietin, dialytic removal of anti-epileptics.
2. Metabolic: hypoglycaemia, hypocalcaemia, hypomagnesemia and hypernatremia.
3. Uremic encephalopathy.

4. Focal neurologic disease: haemorrhage.

5. Other: cardiac arrhythmia and hypertensive encephalopathy.

Treatment may require cessation of dialysis, maintenance of airway, i.v lorazepam and subsequent investigations.

2.2.4 Headache

It is one of the common complications during haemodialysis with a prevalence of 27–73% and consists of bilateral frontal discomfort that is accompanied by nausea and vomiting, but no visual disturbance [11].

Etiopathogenesis is not completely understood.

Management strategy includes:

Optimization of haemodialysis, avoidance of caffeine and blood pressure control.

However, no drugs have been compared in randomized trials to prevent dialysis-related headaches.

2.3 Haematological complication

2.3.1 Intradialytic haemolysis

Acute haemolysis during haemodialysis can be due to variety of causes, which include [12]:

a. Equipment related: faulty tubing, kinking, small size cannula, abnormalities of blood flow and pumps.

b. Toxins: chloramines, copper, zinc, formaldehyde, sodium hypochlorite, etc.

c. Patient related: uremia, infection, lack of erythropoietin, etc.

d. Drugs: aspirin, sulfonamides, penicillins, etc.

Diagnosis is evident with grossly translucent haemolysed blood observed in the tubing.

Evaluation should include, complete blood count, peripheral blood smear, reticulocyte count, haptoglobin, lactate dehydrogenase, coombs test and analysis of water and dialysis equipment.

2.3.2 Haemorrhage

It is associated with intradialytic use of heparin, a common anticoagulant used during haemodialysis. Bleeding can occur from any site like gastrointestinal, pleural, pericardial, retroperitoneal, etc. [13]. diagnosis includes measuring bleeding time despite limitations.

Management includes reversal of precipitating factor, use of erythropoietin stimulating agents, maintaining haematocrit value above 30%, use of i.v DDAVP at 0.3 mcg/kg and infusion of cryoprecipitate as required.

2.4 Pulmonary complications

2.4.1 Dialysis-associated hypoxemia

During dialysis arterial PaO_2 decreases by 5–20 mmHg reaching nadir at 30–60 minutes then resolves within 60–120 minutes after discontinuation of dialysis. This is usually of no significance unless patient has pre-existing cardiopulmonary disease [14].

In high-risk patients, preventive measures include intradialytic use of oxygen, conventional bicarbonate dialysate, and biocompatible membranes. Further optimizing haematocrit and performing sequential isolated UF followed by HD may reduce the likelihood of hypoxemia.

2.5 Technical malfunction

2.5.1 Air embolism

It is a fatal complication, though rare should be identified early and treated accordingly [15].

Most vulnerable source of air entry into extracorporeal circuit includes pre-pump tubing segment. Other sites include glass bottles, air bubbles in dialysate, and uncuff dialysis catheters.

Clinical manifestation depends on position of patient and includes:

- Sitting position, seizure, and coma in absence of chest symptoms.

- Supine position; obstructive shock, dyspnea, dry cough, and chest tightness.

Immediate management includes: clamping the venous blood line, stopping the blood pump, placing the patient in Trendelenburg position, providing CPR if required, aspirating air from right ventricle and/or hyperbaric oxygen therapy as required.

Preventive measures include checking air detecting alarm system prior to initiating haemodialysis, flushing dialysis catheter prior to dialysis, and dialyzer rinsing before use.

2.5.2 Incorrect dialysate composition

Life-threatening electrolyte disturbance can occur due to incorrect mixing and can be corrected by checking composition prior to initiating dialysis it is usually due to human error, however, nowadays there is a machine that automatically changes the mixing ratio of the concentrate until dialysate solution conductivity falls within the set limits [1, 16].

2.5.3 Clotting of dialysis circuit

Clotting of extracorporeal circuit is a common problem encountered during dialysis and warrants thorough evaluation [1].

Various causes are listed below:

1. Technical: inadequate or poor priming technique.
2. Incorrect heparin loading and maintenance.
3. Vascular access related: inadequate flow, excessive access recirculation and frequent interruption of blood flow.

Management includes prompt identification of cause and correcting it.

2.6 Dialysis reaction

Interaction between patients' blood and dialyzer can lead to various adverse reactions [16].

The common dialyzer reactions include:

2.6.1 Type A dialyzer reaction

It was attributed to dialyzer sterilant ethylene oxide, which is rarely used now, and now it is recommended that dialyzers that are validated for re-use should be approved for re-use. The sterilization should be as per the manufacturer's guidance by heat sterilization, gamma radiation or chemicals like formaldehyde, sodium hypochlorite or peracetic acid.

Symptoms usually develop early between 5 and 20 minutes after start of dialysis and include burning throughout the body and access site, dyspnea, chest tightness and angioedema.

Other symptoms like rhinorrhea, lacrimation, cough, pruritis, nausea and vomiting could also be seen.

Management includes cessation of dialysis, drugs like hydrocortisone, antihistamine and epinephrine with or without respiratory support.

Preventive measures include substituting ethylene oxide, biocompatible membranes and discontinuing reprocessing procedures.

2.6.2 Type B dialyzer reaction

It occurs between 20 and 40 minutes after initiation of dialysis.

The cause is attributed to complement activation.

Symptoms include: chest pain and back pain, which subsided with continuation of dialysis.

Preventive measures include automated cleansing of dialyzer and use of non-cellulose dialyzer.

2.6.3 Febrile reactions

It can be due to infection of microbial contamination of the dialysis apparatus.

Treatment: first asses the hemodynamic stability of patient, if the patient is hypotensive administer i.v fluid, cease the UF, discontinue dialysis, give antipyretic and evaluate the potential cause of infection.

Evaluation of dialysate, water source, vascular access. Identify the potential source of infection and treat.

2.7 Miscellaneous complications

2.7.1 Post-dialysis fatigue

It is an ill-defined term, suggesting washed-out feeling or malaise during or after hemodialysis by the patient. It is seen in about one-third of the hemodialysis patients and is multifactorial in origin [17].

Reduced cardiac output, peripheral vascular disease, depression, poor conditioning, post-dialysis hypotension, hypokalemia and hypoglycemia are suggested risk factors.

Management include:

Increasing frequency and duration of dialysis have been suggested to reduce post-dialysis fatigue.

L-carnitine supplementation 20 mg/kg/day has been shown benefit in reducing the recovery time in hemodialysis patients.

Post-dialysis fatigue is associated with an increase risk of mortality, the higher the post-dialysis recovery time the higher the mortality risk.

2.7.2 Pruritis

It is a common and troubling symptom of itching, which patients experience during and after haemodialysis, the symptom of which cannot be attributed to other causes [18].

It has a prevalence of 22–48% in haemodialysis patients.

Cause is often multifactorial and includes: xerosis, hyperparathyroidism, neuropathy, immune dysregulation and inadequate dialysis.

The two major hypotheses of pathogenesis of uremic pruritis include:

1. Opiod hypothesis: it proposes that over-expression of opioid μ receptors in dermal cells and lymphocyte predisposes to uremic pruritis.

2. Immune hypothesis: it proposes that uremic pruritis is an inflammatory state rather than local skin disorder.

Other proposed theories include toxin deposition, based on observation that pruritis was associated with underdialysis and CKD-MBD.

Treatment involves:

a. Optimising dialysis: Achieving dialysis adequacy of Kt/V of >1.2 has been associated with reduced incidence of itching.

   Expanded haemodialysis is a new concept in haemodialysis with medium cut-off membrane, which increases the clearance of middle and large molecules without significant albumin loss, compared to conventional haemodialysis, which clears only small molecules. This might help patients with severe pruritic symptoms and other complications of CKD (**Table 3**) [19].

Molecules	Chemicals	Clinical effect
Small molecule (<500 Da)	Urea, creatinine, uric acid, β-lipoprotein	Uremic toxicity
Middle molecule (500–25 kDa)	β-2-microglobulin, leptin, κ-FLC	Amyloidosis, CV disease, malnutrition.
Large molecule (25–45 kDa)	IL-6, TNF-α, prolactin	Atherosclerosis, CV disease, sepsis, endothelial dysfunction.

Table 3.
Various sizes of uremic toxins and their clinical effect.

b. Optimising CKD-MBD disorder.

a. Skin emollients.

b. Antihistamines like montelukast or cetirizine.

c. Phototherapy: UV B (wavelength 280–315 nm) is effective in treatment of pruritis.

d. Opioid receptor agonist: nalfurafine given iv after HD improved patient experience.

e. Nalfurafine is an orally active kappa opioid receptor agonist which has shown benefit in treatment of uremic pruritis.

f. Gabapentin: given 300 mg after HD was effective in reducing pruritis.

g. Other therapies include capsaicin, long-chain fatty acids and immunosuppressants.

3. Conclusions

The prevalence of common acute complication of haemodialysis is high ranging from 10 to 70%, despite improvements in technology and knowledge of haemodialysis. Hence, we need to identify the complications as early as possible to treat them and apply preventive measures to improve the outcome of the patients.

Acknowledgements

I would like to thank my professors, colleagues and staff and the patients who helped me to gain experience in haemodialysis.

Conflict of interest

None.

Acronyms and abbreviations

CKD	chronic kidney disease
CPR	cardiopulmonary resuscitation
CNS	central nervous system
ESAs	erythropoietin stimulating agents
HD	haemodialysis
IDH	intradialytic hypotension
MAP	mean arterial pressure
MBD	mineral and bone disorder
PD	peritoneal dialysis
RAAS	renin-angiotensin-aldosterone system
RLS	restless leg syndrome
SBP	systolic blood pressure
UF	ultrafiltration

Author details

Saurav Singh Hamal[1*] and Pratima Khadka[2]

1 Department of Nephrology, TUTH, Nepal

2 Department of Pediatrics, Bheri Hospital, Nepal

*Address all correspondence to: sauravkoid@gmail.com

References

[1] Polkinghorne RK, Kerr PG. Comprehensive Clinical Medicine. 6th ed. China: Elsevier; 2019. p. 1090

[2] Kanbay M, Ertuglu LA, Afsar B, et al. An update review of intradialytic hypotension: Concept, risk factors, clinical implications and management. Clinical Kidney Journal. 2020;**3**:981-993

[3] Prasad B, Hemmett J, Suri R. Five things to know about intradialytic hypertension. Canadian Journal of Kidney Health and Disease. 2022;**9**:1-3

[4] Agarwal R, Alborzi P, Satyan S, et al. Dry-weight reduction in hypertensive hemodialysis patients (DRIP): A randomized, controlled trial. Hypertension. 2009;**53**:500-507

[5] Charytan DM, Foley R, McCollough PA, et al. Arrhythmia and sudden cardiac death in hemodialysis patients: Protocol and baseline characteristics of the monitoring in dialysis study. Clinical Journal of the American Society of Nephrology. 2016;**11**:721-734

[6] Ulu MS, Ahsen A. Muscle cramps during hemodialysis. European Journal of General Medicine. 2015;**12**:277-281

[7] Khajehdehi P, Mojerlou M, Behzadi S, et al. A randomized, double-blind, placebo-controlled trial of supplementary vitamins C, E, and their combination for treatment of hemodialysis cramps. Nephrology, Dialysis, Transplantation. 2001;**16**:1448-1451

[8] Kavanagh D, Siddiqui S, Geddes CC. Restless legs syndrome in patients on dialysis. American Journal of Kidney Diseases. 2004;**43**:763-771

[9] Jaber BL, Schiller B, Burkart JM, et al. Impact of short daily hemodialysis on restless legs and sleep disturbances. Journal of American Society Nephrology. 2011;**6**:1049-1056

[10] Gungor O, Aydin Z, Inci A, et al. Seizures in patients with kidney disease: A neglected problem? Nephrology Dial T. 2021;**10**:1-9

[11] Sousa ME, Carrilho AF, Sampaio RP. Dialysis headache: A narrative review. Headache. 2017;**57**:161-164

[12] Tharmaraj D, Kerr PG. Haemolysis in haemodialysis. Néphrologie. 2017;**22**:838-847

[13] Cheung AK. Biocompatibility of hemodialysis membrane. Journal of American Society Nephrology. 1990;**1**:150-161

[14] Cardoso M, Vinay P, Vinet B, et al. Hypoxemia during hemodialysis: A critical review of the facts. American Journal of Kidney Diseases. 1988;**11**:281-297

[15] O'Quin RJ, Laxminarayan S. Venous air embolism. Archives of Internal Medicine. 1982;**142**:2173-2176

[16] Jabel BL, Pereira BJG. Dialysis reactions. Seminars in Dialysis. 1997;**10**:158-165

[17] Jhamb M, Weisbord SD, Steel LJ, et al. Fatigue in patients receiving maintenance dialysis: A review of definitions, measures and contributing factors. American Journal of Kidney Diseases. 2008;**52**:353-365

[18] Ozen N, Cinar FI, Askin D, et al. Uremic pruritis and associated factors in hemodialysis patients: A multi-center

study. Kidney Research Clinical Practise. 2018;**37**:138-147

[19] Jonny J, Teressa M. Expanded hemodialysis: A new concept of renal replacement therapy. Journal of Investigative Medicine. 2022;**2022**:1-4

Chapter 6

Iatrogenic Errors in Hemodialysis Practices

Guled Abdijalil

Abstract

Chronic kidney disease (CKD) and its evolution to end-stage kidney disease (ESKD) are a rapidly increasing global health and healthcare burden . With more than 850 million people suffering from CKD, acute kidney injury, and renal replacement therapy (RRT), the need for hemodialysis (HD) continues to rise worldwide. However, although the safety profile of hemodialysis has been satisfactory over the years, various errors such as dialysis machine errors, dialysate composition errors, and errors in dialysis techniques have been reported, and the treatment has been associated with the highest mortality rates, followed by kidney transplantation and peritoneal dialysis. Consideration of some of these errors could improve safety by facilitating the implementation of preventive measures. The aim of this study was to highpoint some of the important iatrogenic errors encountered during hemodialysis. This review found that common iatrogenic complications during hemodialysis include iatrogenic hypernatremia, iatrogenic iron overload, iatrogenic pseudoaneurysm, iatrogenic cerebral air embolism, iatrogenic infective endocarditis (IE) in Chronic Hemodialysis (CHD) patients, and major bleeding. Adverse effects associated with these complications include interdialytic weight gains, hypertension, cardiovascular events, local pain, neuropathy, distal embolization, and death.

Keywords: hemodialysis, iatrogenic, complications, patient safety, chronic kidney disease

1. Introduction

Chronic kidney disease (CKD) and its evolution to end-stage kidney disease (ESKD) are a rapidly increasing global health and healthcare burden [1]. In 2016, CKD ranked 13th leading cause of death and is projected to be the 5th leading cause of death globally in 2040 [2]. Worldwide, more than 850 million people suffer from CKD, acute kidney injury, and renal replacement therapy (RRT), a figure that is twice the estimated number of individuals with diabetes across the world [3]. Hemodialysis (HD) is the major mode of treatment for RRT worldwide. Advances in hemodialysis machine technology, dialyzers, and consumables have enabled hemodialysis to evolve from a treatment limited to a minority of patients with acute kidney failure in the 1950s to a life-sustaining routine outpatient treatment for multitudes of patients with CKD globally [4, 5].

Although the safety profile of hemodialysis has been satisfactory over the years, various errors such as dialysis machine errors, dialysate composition errors, and errors in dialysis techniques have been reported [6]. Hemodialysis has been associated with the highest mortality rates, followed by kidney transplantation and peritoneal dialysis [7, 8]. Given that hemodialysis patients are a high-risk population group, an error could have catastrophic consequences for such patients [9]. Patient safety during dialysis is thus a critical topic as it is the foundation of high-quality healthcare and minimal patient mortality. Dialysis facilities are complex as they involve providers from numerous disciplines and the use of advanced technology to care for patients with many serious illnesses. As organizations get more complex, the potential for error rises and possible risks need to be identified and prioritized [10].

Errors during dialysis care can result to harm and death. Numerous studies have detailed the increased risk of errors and their unintended consequences among patients undergoing life-sustaining dialysis [11–15]. Some risks are readily apparent in dialysis facilities, with membrane reuse, water quality, and infection control being key areas of safety risk. Other risks may not be as readily apparent, and data-driven efforts have helped to identify and establish safety measures [10]. According to Kliger, (2015), the most common sources of morbidity during dialysis are human factors at the machine interface and suboptimal communication among caregivers. Dialysis machines are seldom a major source of error and morbidity among patients undergoing dialysis. Other causes of possibly reversible adverse medical outcomes during dialysis include hyperkalemia, medication errors, access-related errors, infections, and patient falls [15]. A surveillance report from the United Kingdom over a period of 30 months indicated that there were 31 adverse incidents and five risks reported to UK authorities, of which 42% were from dialysis centers. About 36% of the incidents were due to failure of dialysis techniques or dialysis machine usage, 22% were due to failure of dialysis equipment or disposables, 19% were due to failure of dialysis machines, and 19% were attributed to medication errors [5].

Evidence suggests that attention to some of the highest-risk domains that patients are exposed to could offer insight into processes of care needed to reduce the risk of error and the effect of medical mistakes on patients. This chapter aimed at identifying and describing the type and frequency of medical errors and adverse events in hemodialysis units.

2. Iatrogenic errors in hemodialysis

2.1 Iatrogenic hypernatremia in hemodialysis

Hypernatremia is infrequent in hemodialysis patients and is often iatrogenic when observed. In peritoneal dialysis patients, it is often a result of excessive ultrafiltration. It is critical to be aware of the potential problems associated with dialysate errors, as well as not ignoring the conductivity alarm to ensure that prompt action can be taken to rectify such a situation. Occurrences of hypernatremia errors in dialysate composition have been reported [16–18]. According to Davenport [5], the final dialysate composition is formulated by proportioning the dialysis water with an acid concentrate and a sodium bicarbonate solution. Errors in bicarbonate composition or acid dialysate concentrate can cause hypernatremia [5].

A case report by Kumar et al. [4] showed that a type 2 diabetic patient with hypertension experienced acute hypernatremia leading to altered sensorium during hemodialysis. The possible causes for this case were iatrogenic, improper dialysis concentrate, the underlying disease, or overriding of conductivity alarm. Overriding of the conductivity alarm along with improper dialysis concentrate was concluded to be the most appropriate causes. Similarly, Obialo et al. [6] reported two cases whereby ESKD patients with diabetes mellitus who had been on hemodialysis for 7 and 5 years complained of excess thirst and had poorly controlled blood pressure. Upon investigation, it was discovered that the online conductivity meter on their dialysis machine showed normal readings instead of the actual high readings of high dialysate sodium. Hypernatremia and symptoms resolved completely in both patients on replacement of the dialysis machine.

Different dialysis machines apply different techniques to adjust the final concentration of electrolytes and bicarbonate. Although dialysis machines monitor the final dialysate conductivity, not all machines are equipped with a pH monitor. Also, the range of conductivity permitted differs, hence, some dialysis machines are more dependent on both the healthcare provider correctly inputting the right dialysate composition into the dialysis machine and the dialysate manufacturer providing a reliable product. Incorrect input or supply of different composition can lead to patients dialyzing against inappropriately low or high dialysate sodium [16, 17]. Hypernatremic dialysates lead to increased thirst, interdialytic weight gains, and hypertension [5]. Other forms of dialysate composition errors include machine calibration errors, manufacturing errors, temperature reading errors, and errors in the proportioning system. An incorrect conductivity reading on the other hand can cause patients to dialyze on erroneously low or high dialysate sodium [6].

2.2 Iatrogenic iron overload

Iron overload has for a long time been considered rare in hemodialysis patients especially currently where erythropoiesis-stimulating agents (ESA) are regularly used to manage anemia in hemodialysis patients [19]. Treatment with these agents can, however, cause functional iron deficiency, necessitating iron supplementation [20]. Most studies in the past two decades focused on the detection and management of iron deficiency among dialysis patients. It was not until recently that iron overload among dialysis patients received attention [21]. Iron overload was generally considered to be more prevalent during the pre-ESA era, and anemia was often treated with blood transfusion. Fewer than 10% of patients in this era were dependent on transfusion, but over time, these patients developed iron overload, making this a problematic clinical issue [22].

Although further investigation is needed, a positive correlation has been reported between serum ferritin and LIC determined by MRI T2* and that serum ferritin of more than 290 mcg/L is equivalent to severe iron overload on MRI T2* [23]. A study conducted among Australian dialysis patients with a median ferritin of 782 lg/L by [24] using relaxometry showed that two-thirds of the patients had a hepatic iron overload. In another study, liver iron concentration (LIC) among 119 hemodialysis patients receiving both parenteral iron and ESA was measured by means of T1 and T2* contrast magnetic resonance imaging (MRI) without gadolinium [25]. The findings showed that only 19 out of 119 hemodialysis patients exhibited normal hepatic iron stores, while the rest of the patients (84%) had mild to severe hepatic iron overload. The iron dose infused per month was strongly correlated with both the overall and monthly increase in LIC in 11 patients who were monitored closely during parenteral iron therapy. Additionally, the MRI showed anomalies in the spleen a sign of secondary hemosiderosis in several patients [25]. Reported a case of a 68-year-old woman with CKD receiving dialysis and iron supplementation who presented to the hospital with symptoms whose diagnosis revealed a case of porphyria cutanea tards. Upon examination, extremely high serum ferritin levels (6000 µg/L), suggesting iron overload, were observed. Oral iron supplementation was immediately discontinued, and iron chelators were administered to the patient. After four-month follow-up, normal ferritin level (97.7 µg/L) and improvement in the cutaneous manifestations of porphyria cutanea tarda were observed [26].

Since the body has no natural way to get rid of iron, excessive intravenous iron can lead to iron overload. According to Aldwairi & Yassin [19], excessive iron infusions can result to cardiovascular events and mortality among hemodialysis patients. Excess iron may accumulate in the heart, liver and endocrine organs, leading to cirrhosis of the liver, heart failure, arrhythmia, diabetes mellitus, increased risk of infection and numerous endocrinopathies [27–30]. The adverse effects of iron supplementation can be attributed to the elevated oxidative stress as well as the induction of mononuclear cell adhesion to endothelial cells, which is a critical stage in the pathogenesis of atherosclerosis [31]. Given these findings, there might be a need to revise the guidelines on iron therapy in hemodialysis, especially in terms of the amount of iron infused.

2.3 Iatrogenic pseudoaneurysm

Generally, native autogenous arteriovenous fistula (AVF) is the first choice in vascular access for end-stage renal disease (ESRD), patients who need RRT. This is because fistulas have lower complication rates and better longevity compared to prosthetic grafts [32, 33]. Since the AVF needs time before it can be used, the central venous catheter (CVC) is recommended as the alternative hemodialysis access [34]. In some instances, medical staff and patients usually prefer hemodialysis access with a direct puncture in peripheral vascular while waiting for AVF maturation. A direct puncture and insufficient therapy afterward result in a higher risk of pseudoaneurysm [33]. Iatrogenic pseudoaneurysm (PSA) occurs when the puncture site in an artery fails to heal completely causing a leakage of blood to the surrounding tissue, which manifests in the form of a pulsatile hematoma. It can present as a new thrill, bruit, pulsatile swelling, marked pain or tenderness [35]. The rate of PSA occurrence has been reported at approximately 2–10% [33].

A prospective cross-sectional study conducted by Lone et al. [35] on the characteristics of pseudoaneurysms in North India showed that two of the patients had pseudoaneurysms in relation to arterialized cephalic vein post-radio-cephalic AV fistula at cannulation site for hemodialysis (one of them with multiple pseudoaneurysms along the course of an arterialized cephalic vein), one patient had a pseudoaneurysm linked with brachial artery at brachiocephalic arteriovenous (AV) fistula site for hemodialysis, and another one exhibited pseudoaneurysm in relation to carotid artery after their carotid artery was punctured while placing a central line. Similarly, reported the case of a patient requiring hemodialysis referred for a fistulogram to evaluate his right-arm hemodialysis fistula. Imaging revealed an aneurysmal dilatation of the arteriovenous anastomosis of the right brachial artery and right median cubital vein.

Pseudoaneurysm complications include local pain, neuropathy, distal embolization, rupture, and local skin ischemia. It may also lead to local sepsis and abscess formation, which may rupture and cause hemorrhage [36]. Factors that result in pseudoaneurysms include poor puncture techniques, use of large caliber needles, and premature puncturing of the fistula after surgery [32]. Other factors reported to contribute are catheterization for vascular intervention, arterial gas sampling, penetrating and blunt trauma, and drug abuse [32, 37–39]. The different forms of venous pseudoaneurysm are mainly diagnosed by ultrasound AVF monitoring that is especially important when the pseudoaneurysm is deep and not visible [40]. Treatment options for pseudoaneurysms include surgical repair, endovascular treatment, and minimally invasive percutaneous treatments [41]. In the case of femoral artery pseudoaneurysm, ultrasound-guided manual compression is a well-accepted treatment option, but it is seldom reported in hemodialysis arteriovenous fistula [40].

2.4 Iatrogenic infective endocarditis (IE) in hemodialysis patients

Despite preventive measures implemented by nephrologists, the incidence of IE in CHD remains high. The prevalence of IE in CHD patients is estimated at 2.9% with the incidence being 50–60 times higher than in the general population [40, 42]. The first evidence of IE because of CHD has been described in 1966 and after that, several cases have been reported [40]. A study conducted among French hemodialysis patients showed an overall IE incidence of 2 per 1000 patients, which was 50 times higher than in the general population. The United States healthcare system similarly reported that the incidence of IE among hemodialysis patients was 18 times than that of the general population [43].

It is worth noting that susceptibility to endocarditis in patients undergoing hemodialysis is multifactorial, with numerous factors playing a significant role in the predisposition and development of IE [44]. These factors include those related to the patient's intrinsic susceptibility due to older age and several comorbidities such as hyperuricemia-induced immunosuppression, high exposure to pathogenic microorganisms during hemodialysis sessions following repeated manipulations of their vascular access and the quality of heart valves [44, 45]. The most common location of IE among chronic hemodialysis patients is the left heart and different researchers have reported 80–100% prevalence of left valve involvement. More than 50% of IE cases in CHD are preceded by an episode of bacteremia that originates in more than 70% of cases in a central venous catheter for hemodialysis.

Although international recommendations advocate for use of catheters in less than 10% of patients in a hemodialysis center, this has been difficult to achieve. Catheter-related bacteremia (CRB) is the most common and most dreaded of complications, with an incidence of 2.5–5.5 episodes per 1000 catheter days. CRB is among the highest contributors to IE development and reducing the frequency of CRB would drastically diminish the occurrence of IE.

2.5 Dialysis-induced hypotension (DIH)

Dialysis-induced hypotension (DIH) is one of the most frequent complications in RRT and a very serious clinical problem [46]. Dialysis hypotension occurs in one of three clinical patterns including episodic (acute) hypotension, which involves a sudden drop of systolic blood pressure below 90 mmHg or at least 20 mmHg alongside clinical symptoms, recurrent hypotension, which also involves drops in systolic blood pressure to similar levels as acute hypotension but prevailing in at least 50% of dialysis sessions and chronic hypotension whereby less than 90–100 mmHg interdialytic systolic blood pressure is maintained [47]. Intradialytic hypotension occurs in 15–30% of conventional dialysis treatments and approximately 35% of other techniques such as therapeutic apheresis [46, 48]. The incidence of acute DIH has risen to

50% owing to the increasing number of elder and diabetic patients in the hemodialysis population while that of chronic dialysis hypotension is estimated to occur in 3–5% of dialyzed patients [46].

DIH is usually associated with symptoms such as nausea and vomiting, vertigo, muscle cramps, dyspnea, anxiety, abdominal and chest pain light-headedness, weakness, paleness, and sweating, thus diminishing the quality of life of patients. Further, dialysis hypotension may result in the collapse of the arterial and venous fistula (AVF) and is an independent risk factor for mortality among hemodialysis patients [49]. The pathophysiology of DIH has been reported to be multifactorial and is associated with both host-related factors like cardiovascular diseases and hemodialysis factors like the volume and velocity of the ultrafiltration fluid [48]. The main contributors to hypotension during dialysis include incorrect calculation of ideal weight (dry weight) for the patients leading to high filtration rates, dialysis with acetate buffer, autonomic neuropathy especially among elderly patients with diabetes, non-biocompatible materials used in the production of dialysis equipment, low sodium and high calcium or high magnesium dialysate concentration, chronic inflammation caused by dialysis, and high dialysate temperature [46, 48].

Efficient treatment of DIH is still a great challenge to nephrologists. Sufficient therapy is difficult and needs a multilevel strategy. Nephrology staff and patients need to be well informed regarding the possibilities of hypotension, its symptoms, and its effects on dialysis therapy [50]. Emergency management of DIH includes reduction or cessation of ultrafiltration rate and reduction of blood flow rate. Common measures of long-term treatment and prevention of DIH include accurate determination and frequent evaluation of patients' dry weight, educating patients to avoid excessive interdialytic weight gain, prevention of excess salt and fluid intake (sometimes it is essential to skip or reduce drug dose on the day of dialysis session), ensuring proper dialysis fluid temperature, use of bicarbonate dialysate buffer (instead of acetate) and biocompatible membranes, preventing food intake during dialysis, avoiding the use of low-sodium and low-calcium dialysis fluid, and dose adjustments of anti-hypertensive medications [51, 52].

2.6 Iatrogenic cerebral air embolism

Air embolism is a known iatrogenic clinical problem causing serious morbidity and mortality. It entails the introduction of air into the venous and arterial circulation, which can occur through a myriad of intravascular surgeries and procedures such as hemodialysis [53]. The entrance of air into the systemic veins results in venous air embolism, while entrance into the pulmonary system causes arterial air embolism [54]. Air embolism during renal dialysis is a rare occurrence but potentially catastrophic and often fatal when it occurs [53, 55]. Despite advanced safeguards in procedural techniques and medical hardware, errors may still occur, causing fatal outcomes. Several cases of cerebral embolism during hemodialysis have been reported [55–58].

A case presented by Hysell [57] described a patient with a medical history significant for chronic myeloid leukemia, chronic right foot osteomyelitis, hypertension, and end-stage renal disease on hemodialysis. The patient presented for evaluation of altered mental status alongside acute visual loss after exhibiting symptoms of acute "sleepiness" during dialysis, repetitive speech, and blindness in both eyes upon being aroused. There was no prior history of visual loss and no signs of acute trauma. After examination and considering recent hemodialysis, a head computed tomography

(CT) scan gave findings consistent with air in vascular structures. The patient was placed on 100% oxygen through a nonrebreather and placed in trendelenburg position, and thereafter transferred to a hyperbolic center for definitive management. This case demonstrates an iatrogenic error where the air was introduced into a patient's vascular system during dialysis. In this case, it was found that the dialysate fluid was changed during the dialysis procedure without pausing the dialysis [56].

Air bubbles can be introduced into the dialysis circuit in numerous ways including pre-existing gas bubbles in dialysis tubing and dialyze, pressure or temperature gradients between the patient and the dialysis machine, turbulent blood flow surrounding venous access sites, and introduction of air during connection/disconnection of dialysis tubing [59]. Although there are protocols in place for proper flushing of lines and catheters, as well as patient positioning, the occurrence of air embolism in hemodialysis remains possible and has proven to be lethal when emboli occlude cardiac, neurologic, and pulmonary vasculature. Furthermore, despite being equipped with air traps and ultrasonic detectors, hemodialysis devices are not infallible in filtering microbubbles coming from Luer lock connector tubing or inadequate priming of dialysis hardware [59–61]. The bubbles might move through the circuit without triggering the system alarm, especially when the bubbles have a diameter of less than 50 μL or the flow rates are below the International Electrotechnical Commission infusion pumps and dialysis machines' standard (0.1 ml/kg body weight for bolus infusion or 0.03 ml/kg/minute for continuous infusion) [59, 62].

According to Bessereau [63], long-term data from a tertiary center specializing in managing venous air embolism cases showed a 25% mortality rate for patients affected by air embolus with about 50% of the survivors suffering from neurological sequelae permanently. It is worth noting that diagnosis can be difficult, as only 75% of cerebral air embolism patients will manifest visible air on CT [57]. Given the notoriously dreary consequence of venous air embolism despite aggressive treatment, the importance of proper preventive measures can not be overstated. Cerebral air embolism is deemed an emergency and therapy follow guidelines for other air embolus cases including interruption of the dialysis procedure, efforts to aspirate intravascular gas, external cardiac massage, immediate oxygenation, at best under hyperbaric conditions (HBO) and treatment with benzodiazepines, or barbiturates for patients exhibiting seizures [56, 63, 64]. Additionally, positioning the patient in a head-down trendelenburg position has been suggested, preventing intracardiac air from traveling out to the lungs although some studies have demonstrated a lack of clinical improvement with such exercises. This practice should be avoided in patients with cerebral air embolism as it may potentially exacerbate cerebral edema [54, 57].

Research and development of endovascular therapy as a potential treatment for cerebral air embolism is underway with a single case report documenting the capability of using reperfusion techniques to access affected cerebral vessels, mechanically extracting occluding air bubbles. Moreover, balloon-assisted flow reversal, coupled with suction aspiration, has also been demonstrated [65, 66].

2.7 Major bleeding in hemodialysis

Generally, hemodialysis patients are at a high risk of bleeding due to numerous factors including anemia, uremic platelet dysfunction, and heparin use during dialysis [67]. A retrospective cohort study showed that 1 out of 7 ESRD patients on dialysis experiences a major hemorrhage within 3 years of dialysis initiation [68]. Bleeding in uremia entails an acquired defect of primary hemostasis as a result of platelet

Iatrogenic disease	Causes	Prevention and/or treatment
Iatrogenic hypernatremia in hemodialysis	excessive ultrafiltration Dialysate composition errors Faulty conductivity meter on a dialysis machine	Healthcare providers should correctly input the right dialysate composition into the dialysis machine Supply of reliable products from dialysate manufacturer
Iatrogenic Iron overload	Excessive intravenous iron	Lower use of IV iron products A new therapeutic option has been suggested for compensating iron deficiency linked to hemodialysis and for providing the iron needed for erythropoiesis: Iron administration through the dialysate ferric pyrophosphate citrate (Triferic®) and a ferric citrate-based phosphate binder (Auryxia®)
Iatrogenic pseudoaneurysm	Failure of a peripheral vascular puncture site for hemodialysis to heal completely causes a leakage of blood to the surrounding tissue, which manifests in the form of a pulsatile hematoma	Treatment is via: surgical repair, ultrasound-guided compression repair, endovascular treatment, and minimally invasive percutaneous treatments (coil embolization, thrombin injection)
Iatrogenic infective endocarditis (IE) in chronic hemodialysis patients	Catheter-related bacteremia (CRB) whose risk factors include the following: Hyperuricemia-induced immunosuppression High exposure to pathogenic microorganisms during hemodialysis sessions following repeated manipulations of vascular access and the quality of heart valves	Reducing hospital-acquired bacteremia Antibiotic prophylaxis according to the local guidelines where applicable Good oral hygiene Use of antibacterial coating materials in implantable devices Treatment involves antibiotic therapy and early surgery were required
Dialysis-induced hypotension (DIH)	Incorrect calculation of ideal weight (dry weight) for the patients leading to high filtration rates, Dialysis with acetate buffer Autonomic neuropathy especially among elderly patients with diabetes Non-biocompatible materials used in the production of dialysis equipment Low sodium and high calcium or high magnesium dialysate concentration Chronic inflammation due to dialysis and high dialysate temperature	Accurate determination and frequent evaluation of patients' dry weight Educating patients to avoid excessive interdialytic weight gain Prevention of excess salt and fluid intake Ensuring proper dialysis fluid temperature Use of bicarbonate dialysate buffer (instead of acetate) and biocompatible membranes Preventing food intake during dialysis Avoiding the use of low-sodium and low-calcium dialysis fluid and dose adjustments of anti-hypertensive medications Treatment includes reduction or cessation of ultrafiltration rate and reduction of blood flow rate
Iatrogenic cerebral air embolism	Introduction of air into the venous and arterial circulation due to: pre-existing gas bubbles in dialysis tubing and dialyze Pressure or temperature gradients between the patient and the dialysis machine Turbulent blood flow surrounding venous access sites Introduction of air during connection/disconnection of dialysis tubing	Prevention: proper flushing of lines and catheters and proper patient positioning Treatment involves: interruption of the dialysis procedure, efforts to aspirate intravascular gas, external cardiac massage, and immediate oxygenation, at best under hyperbaric conditions (HBO) Endovascular therapy as a potential treatment for cerebral air embolism is underway

Iatrogenic disease	Causes	Prevention and/or treatment
Major bleeding in hemodialysis	Anemia, uremic platelet dysfunction systemic anticoagulation caused by intermittent administration of heparin	Use of anticoagulation and antiplatelet drugs should be contraindicated for patients already using heparin at every treatment and have known intrinsic platelet dysfunction when receiving dialysis

Table 1.
Summary of iatrogenic complications, their causes, preventive measures and management and treatment.

dysfunction, altered interaction between the platelets and vessel wall and systemic anticoagulation caused by intermittent administration of heparin [67, 68]. In addition to hemostatic changes caused by uremia in hemodialysis patients, hemodialysis therapy itself contributes to various hemostatic changes. These include a decrease in the negative effects on platelet functions of middle molecule uremic toxins, assumed to be eliminated during hemodialysis, coagulation cascade activation due to contact between blood elements and the dialysis membrane, and the effect of anticoagulants used to prevent coagulation resulting from the cascade activation [69].

In conventional hemodialysis, heparin is used to prevent clotting in the extracorporeal circuit by inhibiting the intrinsic coagulation pathway. Although the information on the efficacy of the utilization of antiplatelet and anticoagulation agents among hemodialysis patients is scarce, a few studies have reported that their prescription may cause harm [70]. The systemic anticoagulative effect of heparin presents a bleeding risk. To prevent thrombosis or fistula, health providers may prescribe coumarins and aspirin to hemodialysis patients but these further increase the risk of bleeding. In CKD patients, this risk of bleeding may be worsened by insufficient control of hypertension, diabetic retinopathy, gastrointestinal lesions, and renal cystic disease. For patients without ESRD, antithrombotic agents like oral anticoagulants (OAC) are often administered to prevent stroke in atrial fibrillation, while anti-platelet agents (APA) are indicated for preventing myocardial infarction and cardiovascular death. A study by Elliott [71] showed that in ESRD patients, warfarin doubled the risk of major bleeding. Another study among 255 dialysis patients showed that warfarin increased the risk of bleeding up to four times, while aspirin increased the risk by five times [72]. In addition to its effect on platelet function, it may trigger gastric erosions [72]. These studies emphasize the likelihood that anticoagulation and antiplatelet drugs may have a different risk profile in hemodialysis patients and their use singly or in combination might be contraindicated for patients who are already using heparin at every treatment and have known intrinsic platelet dysfunction when receiving dialysis (**Table 1**) [70].

3. Conclusion

Generally, patients receiving hemodialysis often experience the low health-related quality of life (HRQOL), including pain, fatigue and emotional distress. It is critical, therefore, to ensure patient safety during hemodialysis to prevent morbidity and mortality as a result of iatrogenic complications. In this study, some of the identified common errors during hemodialysis include iatrogenic hypernatremia in hemodialysis, iatrogenic iron overload, iatrogenic pseudoaneurysm, iatrogenic infective endocarditis in chronic hemodialysis patients, iatrogenic cerebral air embolism, and major bleeding. Continuous monitoring of equipment is essential within hemodialysis services so that measures can be taken to minimize such occurrences. It is also recommended that duly validated protocols that define roles and organize the processes related to patient care are developed, in addition to continuous education for professionals.

Conflict of interest

The authors declare no conflict of interest or delete this entire section.

Author details

Guled Abdijalil[1,2]

1 Department of Nephrology, Shaoxing People's Hospital (Shaoxing Hospital Zhejiang University School of Medicine), Shaoxing, Zhejiang, China

2 School of Medicine, Shaoxing University, Shaoxing, Zhejiang, China

*Address all correspondence to: guledabdijalil@gmail.com

References

[1] Thurlow JS, Joshi M, Yan G, Norris KC, Agodoa LY, Yuan CM, et al. Global epidemiology of end-stage kidney disease and disparities in kidney replacement therapy. American Journal of Nephrology. 2021;**52**(2):98-107 [Internet] [cited 2022 Nov 15] Available from: https://www.karger.com/Article/FullText/514550

[2] de Ferreira ES, Moreira TR, da Silva RG, da Costa GD, da Silva LS, de Cavalier SBO, et al. Survival and analysis of predictors of mortality in patients undergoing replacement renal therapy: A 20-year cohort. BMC Nephrology 2020;21(1):1-14

[3] Jager KJ, Kovesdy C, Langham R, Rosenberg M, Jha V, Zoccali C. A single number for advocacy and communication-worldwide more than 850 million individuals have kidney diseases. Kidney International. 2019;**96**(5):1048-1050 [Internet] [cited 2022 Nov 15] Available from: http://www.ncbi.nlm.nih.gov/pubmed/31582227

[4] Kumar A, Singh R, Vikrant S. Iatrogenic hypernatremia; still not uncommon. International Journal of Clinical Skills. 2022;**16**(6):246 [Internet] [cited 2022 Nov 16] Available from: https://www.ijocs.org/clinical-journal/iatrogenic--hypernatremia-still-not-uncommon-15433.html

[5] Davenport A. Complications of hemodialysis treatments due to dialysate contamination and composition errors. Hemodialysis International. 2015;**19**:S30-S33 [Internet] [cited 2022 Nov 16] Available from: https://onlinelibrary.wiley.com/doi/full/10.1111/hdi.12350

[6] Obialo CI, John S, Bashir K. Iatrogenic hypernatremia in hemodialysis patients: A result of erroneous online conductivity monitor and conductivity meter reading. Hemodialysis International. 2017;**21**(4):E73-E75 [Internet] [cited 2022 Nov 17] Available from: https://onlinelibrary.wiley.com/doi/full/10.1111/hdi.12546

[7] Kainz A, Berner C, Ristl R, Simon A, Stamm T, Zitt E, et al. Sex-specific analysis of haemodialysis prevalence, practices and mortality over time: The Austrian dialysis registry from 1965 to 2014. Nephrology, Dialysis, Transplantation. 2019;**34**(6):1026-1035 [Internet] [cited 2022 Nov 15] Available from: https://pubmed.ncbi.nlm.nih.gov/30476247/

[8] Carrero JJ, Hecking M, Chesnaye NC, Jager KJ. Sex and gender disparities in the epidemiology and outcomes of chronic kidney disease. Nature Reviews. Nephrology. 2018;**14**(3):151-164 [Internet] [cited 2022 Nov 15] Available from: https://pubmed.ncbi.nlm.nih.gov/29355169/

[9] Arenas Jiménez MD, Ferre G, Álvarez-Ude F. Strategies to increase patient safety in haemodialysis: Application of the modal analysis system of errors and effects (FEMA system). Nefrologist (English Ed). 2017;**37**(6):608-621 [Internet] [cited 2022 Nov 17] Available from: https://www.revistanefrologia.com/en-strategies-increase-patient-safety-in-articulo-S2013251417301955

[10] Garrick R, Kliger A, Stefanchik B. Patient and facility safety in hemodialysis: Opportunities and strategies to develop a culture of safety. Clinical Journal of the American Society of Nephrology. 2012;**7**(4):680-688 [Internet] [cited 2022 Nov 14] Available

from: https://cjasn.asnjournals.org/content/7/4/680

[11] Ellingson KD, Palekar RS, Lucero CA, Kurkjian KM, Chai SJ, Schlossberg DS, et al. Vascular access hemorrhages contribute to deaths among hemodialysis patients. Kidney International. 2012;**82**(6):686-692 [Internet] [cited 2022 Nov 14] Available from: https://pubmed.ncbi.nlm.nih.gov/22695325/

[12] Camins BC. Prevention and treatment of hemodialysis-related bloodstream infections. Seminars in Dialysis. 2013;**26**(4):476-481 [Internet] [cited 2022 Nov 14] Available from: https://pubmed.ncbi.nlm.nih.gov/23859190/

[13] Ward RA, Ronco C. Improvements in technology: A path to safer and more effective hemodialysis. Blood Purification. 2009;**27**(1):6-10 [Internet] [cited 2022 Nov 14] Available from: https://pubmed.ncbi.nlm.nih.gov/19169010/

[14] Kliger AS. Patient safety in the dialysis facility. Blood Purification. 2006;**24**(1):19-21 [Internet] [cited 2022 Nov 14] Available from: https://pubmed.ncbi.nlm.nih.gov/16361835/

[15] Kliger AS. Maintaining safety in the dialysis facility. Clinical Journal of the American Society of Nephrology. 2015;**10**(4):688-695 [Internet] [cited 2022 Nov 14] Available from: https://cjasn.asnjournals.org/content/10/4/688

[16] Bhosale GP, Shah VR. Saudi journal of kidney diseases and transplantation. Saudi Journal of Kidney Diseases and Transplantation. 2015;**26**(1):107 [Internet] [cited 2022 Nov 16] Available from: https://www.sjkdt.org/article.asp?issn=1319-2442;year=2015;volume=26;issue=1;spage=107;epage=110;aulast=Bhosale

[17] Sandhu E, Crawford C, Davenport A. Weight gains and increased blood pressure in outpatient hemodialysis patients due to change in acid dialysate concentrate supplier. The International Journal of Artificial Organs. 2012;**35**(9):642-647 [Internet] [cited 2022 Nov 16] Available from: https://journals.sagepub.com/doi/10.1177/039139881203500903

[18] Williams DJ, Harding K, Woolfson RG, Mansell MA, Jugumauth J. Acute hypernatraemia during bicarbonate-buffered haemodialysis. Nephrology, Dialysis, Transplantation. 1994;**9**(8):1170-1173 [Internet] [cited 2022 Nov 17] Available from: https://pubmed.ncbi.nlm.nih.gov/7800220/

[19] Aldwairi MM, Yassin MA. Iatrogenic iron overload in an end stage renal disease patient. Case Reports in Oncology. 2020;**13**(2):760-763

[20] Rostoker G, Vaziri ND, Fishbane S. Iatrogenic iron overload in dialysis patients at the beginning of the 21st century. Drugs. 2016;**76**(7):741-757 [Internet] [cited 2022 Nov 17] Available from: https://pubmed.ncbi.nlm.nih.gov/27091216/

[21] Vaziri ND. Epidemic of iron overload in dialysis population caused by intravenous iron products: A plea for moderation. The American Journal of Medicine. 2012;**125**(10):951-952 [Internet] [cited 2022 Nov 24] Available from: https://pubmed.ncbi.nlm.nih.gov/22795817/

[22] Coyne DW. Iron overload in dialysis patients: Rust or bust? Kidney International Reports. 2017;**2**(6):995-997 [Internet] [cited 2022 Nov 28] Available from: http://www.kireports.org/article/S2468024917303728/fulltext

[23] Ghoti H, Rachmilewitz EA, Simon-Lopez R, Gaber R, Katzir Z, Konen E, et al. Evidence for tissue iron overload in long-term hemodialysis patients and the impact of withdrawing parenteral iron. European Journal of Haematology. 2012;**89**(1):87-93 [Internet] [cited 2022 Nov 28] Available from: https://pubmed.ncbi.nlm.nih.gov/22435497/

[24] Ferrari P, Kulkarni H, Dheda S, Betti S, Harrison C, St Pierre TG, et al. Serum iron markers are inadequate for guiding iron repletion in chronic kidney disease. Clinical Journal of the American Society of Nephrology. 2011;**6**(1):77 [Internet] [cited 2022 Nov 24] Available from: http://pmc/articles/PMC3022252/

[25] Rostoker G, Griuncelli M, Loridon C, Couprie R, Benmaadi A, Bounhiol C, et al. Hemodialysis-associated Hemosiderosis in the era of erythropoiesis-stimulating agents: A MRI study. The American Journal of Medicine. 2012;**125**(10):991-999 [Internet] [cited 2022 Nov 28] Available from: https://pubmed.ncbi.nlm.nih.gov/22998881/

[26] AlGahtani FH, Stuckey R, Alqahtany FS. Secondary hemosiderosis presented by porphyria cutanea tarda in a kidney dialysis patient: A case report. SAGE Open Medical Case Reports. 2020;**8**:2050313X2090781 [Internet] [cited 2022 Nov 28] Available from: https://journals.sagepub.com/doi/full/10.1177/2050313X20907815

[27] Soliman AT, Yassin M, Majuid NMSA, Sabt A, Abdulrahman MO, De SV. Cortisol response to low dose versus standard dose (back-to-back) adrenocorticotrophic stimulation tests in children and young adults with thalassemia major. Indian. Journal of Endocrinology and Metabolism. 2013;**17**(6):1046 [Internet] [cited 2022 Nov 24] Available from: http://pmc/articles/PMC3872683/

[28] Kuo KL, Hung SC, Lin YP, Tang CF, Lee TS, Lin CP, et al. Intravenous Ferric Chloride Hexahydrate Supplementation Induced Endothelial Dysfunction and Increased Cardiovascular Risk among Hemodialysis Patients. PLoS One. 2012;**7**(12):1-11. DOI: 10.1371/journal.pone.0050295

[29] Sanctis V De, Elsedfy H, Soliman AT, Elhakim IZ, Pepe A, Kattamis C, et al. Acquired Hypogonadotropic Hypogonadism (AHH) in Thalassaemia Major Patients: An Underdiagnosed Condition? Mediterranean Journal of Hematology and Infectious Diseases. 2016;**8**(1):1-9. DOI: 10.4084/MJHID.2016.001

[30] Ali M, Okar L, Iqbal P, Yassin, MA. Iatrogenic Iron Overload in a Patient With Chronic Kidney Disease: Is There a Correlation Between Serum Ferritin and Liver Iron Concentration Determined by MRI T2*? Cureus. 2020;**12**(6):1-6. DOI: 10.7759/cureus.8914

[31] Rostoker G, Vaziri ND. Iatrogenic iron overload and its potential consequences in patients on hemodialysis. Presse Médicale. 2017;**46**(12 Pt 2):e312-e328 [Internet] [cited 2022 Nov 24] Available from: https://pubmed.ncbi.nlm.nih.gov/29153377/

[32] Wang A, Silberzweig JE. Brachial artery Pseudoaneurysms caused by inadvertent hemodialysis access needle punctures. American Journal of Kidney Diseases. 2009;**53**(2):351-354 [Internet] [cited 2022 Nov 29] Available from: http://www.ajkd.org/article/S0272638608012468/fulltext

[33] Sulistyaningsih NK, Lie ZY, Limanto DH. Iatrogenic pseudoaneurysm as a complication of hemodialysis

vascular access : A descriptive study. Journal of Indonesia Vascular Access. 2022;**2**(2):25-28

[34] Ikizler TA, Burrowes JD, Byham-Gray LD, Campbell KL, Carrero JJ, Chan W, et al. KDOQI clinical practice guideline for nutrition in CKD: 2020 update. American Journal of Kidney Diseases. 2020;**76**(3 Suppl 1):S1-S107 [Internet] [cited 2022 Nov 29] Available from: https://pubmed.ncbi.nlm.nih.gov/32829751/

[35] Lone H, Ganaie FA, Lone GN, Dar AM, Bhat MA, Singh S, et al. Characteristics of Pseudoaneurysms in northern India; risk analysis, clinical profile, surgical management and outcome. Bull Emerg. Trauma. 2015;**3**(2):59 [Internet] [cited 2022 Nov 29] Available from: http://pmc/articles/PMC4771268/

[36] Sirvent AE, Enríquez R, Reyes A, Martínez D. Delayed presentation of femoral pseudoaneurysm after hemodialysis catheter insertion procedure. Nefrologist (English Ed). 2008;**28**(6):654-655 [Internet] [cited 2022 Nov 29] Available from: https://www.revistanefrologia.com/en-delayed-presentation-femoral-pseudoaneurysm-after-articulo-X2013251408004417

[37] Yetkin U, Gurbuz A. Post-traumatic Pseudoaneurysm of the brachial artery and its surgical treatment. Texas Heart Institute Journal. 2003;**30**(4):293 [Internet] [cited 2022 Nov 29] Available from: http://pmc/articles/PMC307714/

[38] Yildirim S, Nursal TZ, Yildirim T, Tarim A, Caliskan K. Brachial artery Pseudoaneurysm: A rare complication after Haemodialysis therapy. Acta Chirurgica Belgica. 2005;**105**(2):190-193 [Internet] [cited 2022 Nov 29] Available from: https://www.tandfonline.com/doi/abs/10.1080/00015458.2005.11679697

[39] Siu WT, Kwok KY, Cheung HYS, Law BKB, Chung NT, Yang GPC, et al. Management of brachial artery pseudoaneurysms secondary to drug abuse. Annals of Vascular Surgery. 2005;**19**(5):657-661 [Internet] [cited 2022 Nov 29] Available from: https://pubmed.ncbi.nlm.nih.gov/16096861/

[40] Rahil MA. Successful treatment of a venous pseudoaneurysm in a brachiobasilic fistula using ultrasound-guided manual compression: Two case reports. Journal of Ultrasound. 2019;**22**(3):345-347 [Internet] [cited 2022 Nov 29] Available from: http://pmc/articles/PMC6704213/

[41] Okwuonu CG, Ojeh-Oziegbe O, Adejumo O, Iyawe I. Iatrogenic femoral artery pseudoaneurysm complicating vascular access for haemodialysis in a patient with end-stage renal disease; unexpected occurrence after a common procedure. Journal of Medicine Tropical. 2016;**18**(2):116 [Internet] [cited 2022 Nov 29] Available from: https://www.jmedtropics.org/article.asp?issn=2276-7096;year=2016;volume=18;issue=2;spage=116;epage=118;aulast=Okwuonu

[42] Oullaï A, Cubilier E, Salaouatchi MT, Taghavi M, Zouggari Y, Nortier J, et al. Iatrogenic infective endocarditis in hemodialysis patients: A case report and review of the literature. Case Reports in Nephrology. 2022;**2022**(8500299):1-6. DOI: 10.1155/2022/8500299

[43] Sadeghi M, Behdad S, Shahsanaei F. Infective endocarditis and its short and long-term prognosis in hemodialysis patients: A systematic review and meta-analysis. Current Problems in Cardiology. 2021;**3**(100680):1-13. DOI: 10.1016/j.cpcardiol.2020.100680

[44] Bentata Y. Physiopathological approach to infective endocarditis in chronic hemodialysis patients: Left

heart versus right heart involvement. Renal Failure. 2017;**39**(1):432-439 [Internet] [cited 2022 Nov 30] Available from: https://pubmed.ncbi.nlm.nih.gov/28335676/

[45] Vaziri ND, Pahl MV, Crum A, Norris K. Effect of uremia on structure and function of immune system. Journal of Renal Nutrition. 2012;**22**(1):149 [Internet] [cited 2022 Nov 30] Available from: http://pmc/articles/PMC3246616/

[46] Sulowicz W, Radziszewski A. Pathogenesis and treatment of dialysis hypotension. Kidney International. 2006;**70**(SUPPL. 104):S36-S39

[47] Dheenan S, Henrich WL. Preventing dialysis hypotension: A comparison of usual protective maneuvers. Kidney International. 2001;**59**(3):1175-1181

[48] Noshad H, Ghorbani R, Herizchi S, Shayan SK, Ghamari B, Shayan FK. Sertraline prevents hypotension during hemodialysis: A randomized clinical trial. Nephrourology Monthly. 2018;**10**(3):1-5. DOI: 10.5812/numonthly.66060

[49] Shoji T, Tsubakihara Y, Fujii M, Imai E. Hemodialysis-associated hypotension as an independent risk factor for two-year mortality in hemodialysis patients. Kidney International. 2004;**66**(3):1212-1220

[50] Hossli SM. Clinical management of intradialytic hypotension: Survey results. Nephrology Nursing Journal. 2005;**32**(3):287-291 quiz 292. [Internet] [cited 2022 Dec 3] Available from: https://pubmed.ncbi.nlm.nih.gov/16035470/

[51] Palmer BF, Henrich WL. Recent advances in the prevention and Management of Intradialytic Hypotension. Journal of American Society of Nephrology. 2008;**19**(1):8-11 [Internet] [cited 2022 Dec 3] Available from: https://jasn.asnjournals.org/content/19/1/8

[52] Assimon MM, Flythe JE. Intradialytic blood pressure abnormalities: The highs, the lows, and all that lies between. American Journal of Nephrology. 2015;**42**(5):337 [Internet] [cited 2022 Dec 3] Available from: http://pmc/articles/PMC4761237/

[53] Hassen FM, Dalla AS, Ayed S, Tilouche N, Ali BS, Gharbi R, et al. Delayed treatment of iatrogenic cerebral air embolism with hyperbaric oxygen. Trends in Anaesthesia and Critical Care. 2013;**3**(5):289-290. [Internet]:. DOI: 10.1016/j.tacc.2013.03.004

[54] Wong SSM, Kwaan HC, Ing TS. Venous air embolism related to the use of central catheters revisited: With emphasis on dialysis catheters. Clinical Kidney Journal. 2017;**10**(6):797 [Internet] [cited 2022 Dec 7] Available from: http://pmc/articles/PMC5716215/

[55] Monnell K, Varshney A, Moore B. Stroke due to hemodialysis-associated air embolism. Practical Neurology. 2021:56-59

[56] Lau L, London K. Cortical blindness and altered mental status following routine hemodialysis, a case of iatrogenic cerebral air embolism. Case rep. Emergency Medicine. 2018;**2018**:1-4 [Internet] [cited 2022 Dec 7] Available from: http://pmc/articles/PMC5872667/

[57] Hysell MK. Cerebral air embolism after hemodialysis. The Journal of Emergency Medicine. 2015;**49**(1):e27-e28. [Internet]:. DOI: 10.1016/j.jemermed.2014.12.071

[58] Wesley Ely E, Duncan Hite R, Baker AM, Johnson MM, Bowton DL, Haponik EF. Venous air embolism

from central venous catheterization: A need for increased physician awareness. Critical Care Medicine. 1999;**27**(10):2113-2117 [Internet] [cited 2022 Dec 7] Available from: https://pubmed.ncbi.nlm.nih.gov/10548191/

[59] Barak M, Nakhoul F, Katz Y. Pathophysiology and clinical implications of microbubbles during hemodialysis. Seminars in Dialysis. 2008;**21**(3):232-238 [Internet] [cited 2022 Dec 7] Available from: https://pubmed.ncbi.nlm.nih.gov/18363602/

[60] Mishra R, Reddy P, Khaja M. Fatal cerebral air embolism: A case series and literature review. Case reports. Critical Care. 2016;**2016**:1-4 [Internet] [cited 2022 Dec 7] Available from: http://pmc/articles/PMC5011199/

[61] Forsberg U, Jonsson P, Stegmayr C, Stegmayr B. Microemboli, developed during haemodialysis, pass the lung barrier and may cause ischaemic lesions in organs such as the brain. Nephrology, Dialysis, Transplantation. 2010;**25**(8):2691-2695 [Internet] [cited 2022 Dec 7] Available from: https://pubmed.ncbi.nlm.nih.gov/20305135/

[62] Stegmayr B. Air contamination during hemodialysis should be minimized. Hemodialysis International. 2017;**21**(2):168-172 [Internet] [cited 2022 Dec 7] Available from: https://pubmed.ncbi.nlm.nih.gov/27576675/

[63] Bessereau J, Genotelle N, Chabbaut C, Huon A, Tabah A, Aboab J, et al. Long-term outcome of iatrogenic gas embolism. Intensive Care Medicine. 2010;**36**(7):1180-1187 [Internet] Available from: http://link.springer.com/10.1007/s00134-010-1821-9

[64] Schlimp CJ, Loimer T, Rieger M, Schmidts MB, Lederer W. Pathophysiological mechanism and immediate treatment of retrograde cerebral venous air embolism. Intensive Care Medicine. 2006;**32**(6):945-945 [Internet] [cited 2022 Dec 7] Available from: https://link.springer.com/article/10.1007/s00134-006-0149-y

[65] Belton PJ, Nanda A, Alqadri SL, Khakh GS, Chandrasekaran PN, Newey C, et al. Paradoxical cerebral air embolism causing large vessel occlusion treated with endovascular aspiration. BML Case Reports. 2016;**2016**:bcr2016012535 [Internet] [cited 2022 Dec 7] Available from: http://pmc/articles/PMC4964109/

[66] Kalani MYS, Park MS, Kilburg C, Taussky P. Cerebral air embolism treated with endovascular flow reversal and suction aspiration. Interdisciplinary Neurosurgery. 2017;**10**:17-19 [Internet] [cited 2022 Dec 7] Available from: https://linkinghub.elsevier.com/retrieve/pii/S2214751917300348

[67] Limdi NA, Beasley TM, Baird MF, Goldstein JA, McGwin G, Arnett DK, et al. Kidney function influences warfarin responsiveness and hemorrhagic complications. Journal of American Society of Nephrology. 2009;**20**(4):912 [Internet] [cited 2022 Dec 8] Available from: http://pmc/articles/PMC2663833/

[68] Sood MM, Bota SE, McArthur E, Kapral MK, Tangri N, Knoll G, et al. The three-year incidence of major hemorrhage among older adults initiating chronic dialysis. Canadian Journal of Kidney Health and Disease. 2014;**1**(1):21 [Internet] [cited 2022 Dec 7] Available from: http://pmc/articles/PMC4349720/

[69] Ozkan G, Ulusoy S. Bleeding diathesis in hemodialysis patients. In: Hemodialysis [Internet]. London, UK, London, UK: InTech; 2013. pp. 60-70 [cited 2022 Dec 8] Available from:

https://www.intechopen.com/state.item.id

[70] Chan KE, Lazarus JM, Thadhani R, Hakim RM. Anticoagulant and antiplatelet usage associates with mortality among hemodialysis patients. Journal of American Society of Nephrology. 2009;**20**(4):872-881 [Internet] Available from: https://jasn.asnjournals.org/lookup/doi/10.1681/ASN.2008080824

[71] Elliott MJ, Zimmerman D, Holden RM. Warfarin anticoagulation in hemodialysis patients: A systematic review of bleeding rates. American Journal of Kidney Diseases. 2007;**50**(3):433-440 [Internet] [cited 2022 Dec 8] Available from: https://pubmed.ncbi.nlm.nih.gov/17720522/

[72] Holden RM, Harman GJ, Wang M, Holland D, Day AG. Major bleeding in hemodialysis patients. Clinical Journal of the American Society of Nephrology. 2008;**3**(1):105 [Internet] [cited 2022 Dec 7] Available from: http://pmc/articles/PMC2390984/

Chapter 7

Hyporesponsiveness to Erythropoietin-Stimulating Agents: Possible Solutions

Ahmed Yasin and Nayer Omran

Abstract

Almost 80% of dialysis patients have anemia of different severity, with its pathogenesis of multifactorial nature. Relative insufficiency of erythropoietin leading to hyperproliferative erythropoiesis is considered the main underlying cause. Management of anemia has several therapeutic implications, including reasonable quality of life and avoidance of repeated blood transfusions, among others. Optimal maintenance of hemoglobin target levels is not easy, even with the implementation of different therapeutic options, including erythropoietin-stimulating agents (ESAs). Approximately 5–10% of patients are not responding adequately, despite incremental dosing of ESA therapy. That inadequate response has multiple heterogeneous causes, making anemia management rather difficult. Hyporesponsiveness to ESAs is a challenge requiring a proper approach.

Keywords: dialysis, Anemia, erythropoiesis stimulating agents, hyporesponsiveness, resistance

1. Introduction

According to World Health Organization (WHO), anemia is defined as a Hb level < 13 m/dl in adult males and postmenopausal females, while it is there if Hb levels <12 gm/dl for premenopausal females [1]. Renal anemia is a frequent complication in chronic kidney disease (CKD) patients with worse outcomes of morbidity and mortality [2, 3]. Its severity increases with progressive loss of kidney function, as around 90% of erythropoietin (EPO) is produced by the kidneys [4]. While almost 5% of CKD stage III patients have anemia, approximately 95% of hemodialysis patients develop a certain degree of anemia [5]. Several causative factors are included in the pathogenesis of anemia in CKD patients, mainly the decreased production of EPO [6]. Following the US Food and Drug Administration's approval of recombinant human EPO (rhuEPO) in 1989, the introduction of ESAs was a real revolution in renal anemia management [7]. More than 85% of hemodialysis patients were treated with ESA, according to USRDS 2020 Annual Data report. However, inadequate response to ESA therapy was reported in 5–10% of cases [8].

IntechOpen

2. Definitions

2.1 Hyporesponsiveness vs. resistance

The term hyporesponsiveness looks preferable to the term resistance for its more accuracy as a reduced response to ESA therapy is relative in most cases. So, the word hyporesponsiveness describes the use of higher than usual ESA doses without reaching Hb target levels OR the need for incremental ESA doses to keep target Hb levels [9].

According to KDIGO 2012 guidelines, ESA hyporesponsiveness denotes no increase in Hb following 1 month of weight-based dosing (initial type) and/or the need for two increments in ESA dose up to 50% more than the previous dose for achieving stable Hb levels(subsequent type) [10].

According to European Best Practice guidelines (2004), the maximum dose of EPO is 300 units/kg/week and 1.2 mcg/kg/week for darbepoetin alfa [11].

The ideal Hb level for hemodialysis patients is not well-defined. An accepted practice is to have maintenance of Hb target level between 10 and 11.5 gm/dL. This goes in harmony with KDIGO 2012 guidelines.

2.2 ESA resistance index (ERI)

It is a mathematical representation of the complex relationship between the targeted Hb level and the required ESA dose. It is calculated as the ratio between the average weekly ESA dose/kg body weight and Hb (g/dl) level. Elevated ERI is suggested as a possible clue for modifiable causative factors underlying ESA hyporesponsiveness [12].

3. Epidemiology

The incidence of ESA hyporesponsiveness in hemodialysis patients differs from one country to another, ranging from 7.3 to 17.6%, with more prevalence compared with patients on peritoneal dialysis. ESA hyporesponsiveness was reported in 12.5% of hemodialysis patients and was strongly associated with higher mortality, iron and ESA use, and lower Hb levels. Around 15% of hemodialysis patients requiring high ESA doses have 50% consumption of total ESA therapy costs [13].

4. Etiology

Causes of anemia of ESA hyporesponsiveness are broadly related to three main categories: namely iron deficiency, inflammatory conditions, and bone marrow suppression. A summary of these causes is shown in **Table 1**.

4.1 Iron deficiency

It is considered the most common cause of ESA hyporesponsiveness [14]. Iron deficiency may be absolute or functional type, which is more common. The absolute type is characterized by severely deficient or lacking iron storage, mainly due to blood

Frequent	Less frequent	Unknown
Iron deficiency	Hemorrhage, hemolysis	No cause could be found in one-third of the cases
Inflammation/infection	Hyperparathyroidism	
Inadequate dialysis	Vit. B 12, folate deficiency	
	Bone marrow suppression	
	Pure red cell aplasia	
	Aluminum toxicity	
	Carnitine deficiency	
	Angiotensin-converting enzyme inhibitors	
	ESA subcutaneous administration with obesity	

Table 1.
Summary of causes of ESA hyporesponsiveness.

loss. Usually, transferrin saturation (TSAT)% is less than or equal to 20% with serum ferritin less than 200 ng/mL.

The functional type has normal iron storage with diminished iron availability for erythropoiesis. It is associated with low TSAT % and normal/high ferritin levels. Functional iron deficiency is further divided into two subtypes: the first is related to ESA therapy itself, and the second is attributed to anemia of chronic disease.

Measurement of red blood cells Hb content could be better for the assessment of functional iron deficiency and possible response to iron therapy. This can be achieved through the measurement of hypochromic red blood cell (HRCs) percentage, threshold value more than 6%, and reticulocyte Hb content (CHr); threshold value less than 29 pg., according to NICE guidelines, 2016 [15].

The HRCs % and CHr are more widely used in Europe than in the United States.

In cases with ESA-induced iron deficiency, the response can occur to IV iron administration and concurrent increase of ESA dose together with a resulting decrease of ferritin levels. Conversely, in patients with anemia of chronic disease, IV iron administration will not improve erythropoiesis and will be associated with a progressive increase in ferritin levels [16].

4.2 Inflammation

Chronic inflammatory status is common in hemodialysis patients and is considered a major cause of ESA hyporesponsiveness. Inhibition of production leads to hypoproliferative anemia of chronic disease. Bone marrow and impairment of EPO erythropoiesis renal patient-related specific underlying causes of chronic inflammation include dialysis catheter-related infection, infected or nonfunctioning arteriovenous graft, failed renal allograft, or uremic toxins. Other causes include malignancies, chronic infections, autoimmune disorders, or periodontal disease. Systemic inflammation affecting the immune system function can be a sequence of gut microbiota dysbiosis. IL-6 works in the opposite direction of EPO regarding its effect on bone marrow proliferation. Serum levels of both IL-6 and TNF-alpha are directly related to ESA dose in hemodialysis patients [17–19].

4.3 Inadequate dialysis

Uremic toxins can cause ESA hyporesponsiveness through nonselective bone marrow suppression or through selective suppression of erythroid colony-forming units. Accumulation of quinolinic acid in renal failure leads to inhibition of EPO gene expression, possibly mediated by hypoxia-inducible factor (HIF)1 alfa. Other substances like indoxyl sulfate (IS) and indoxyl glucuronide can suppress transcriptional HIF-1 alfa activity leading to inappropriate EPO production. Dialysis dose should be monitored in malfunctioning dialysis catheters and in fistula with lower blood flow rates. The chronic inflammatory state can occur in hemodialysis patients due to low-level endotoxin and bacterial contamination of dialysis water. This was confirmed through the beneficial effect of using ultrapure water. Based on large randomized clinical trials, the use of high-flux and online treatments, though supposed better removal of large and middle molecules, was not associated with a significant effect on anemia and ESA requirements.

With high predialysis hematocrit values or slow blood flow of vascular access, red blood cell damage can occur due to shear stress and high pressure in dialyzer capillaries.

It was suggested that the use of mixed pre- and postdilution hemodiafiltration (HDF) might be preferred to postdilution HDF through avoidance of progressive hemoconcentration. However, this hypothesis needs further confirmation. There is no clear evidence supporting the beneficial effect of increasing dialysis frequency per se regarding ESA hyporesponsiveness [20–22].

Efforts to improve dialysis quality have led to the development of a novel class of dialysis membranes; called medium cut-off (MCO) with molecular weight cut-off (MWCO) close to MW of albumin and very high retention onset (HRO) [23]. Recently, these membranes are called HRO membranes. They are made of polyarylethersulfone/polyvinylpyrrolidone with a mean pore radius of 5 nm, in between high-flux and high cut-off (HCO) membranes. They are designed to enhance the clearance of molecules larger than B2-microglobulin with the ability of albumin retention. In addition, the internal diameters of the fibers are reduced to increase blood compartment resistance and enhance dialyzer internal filtration and back-filtration. The resulting convection is comparable to that of classical high flux membranes, with effective removal of middle and large molecules without fluid substitution. Using this novel class of dialyzers, HRO is called expanded hemodialysis (EHDx).

EHDx has improved response to ESA therapy in comparison with the use of a high-flux (HF) dialyzer. That effect was attributed to the superior removal of inflammatory cytokines with better iron metabolism in a hepcidin-independent mechanism. More middle-molecule uremic toxins clearance with more reduction of TNF-alfa was achieved with the use of MCO dialyzers than with HF dialyzers. Additionally, high-flux dialysis did not show superiority to low-flux dialysis in improving ESA hyporesponsiveness [24]. In a comprehensive systematic review and meta-analysis study, it was found that EHDx showed safety regarding albumin loss in dialysate and back-filtration of endotoxins. Moreover, EHDx proved effective clearance of middle and large uremic toxin molecules in comparison with high-flux hemodialysis and online HDF with potential anti-inflammatory activity as well [25, 26].

4.4 Aluminum toxicity

Although rarely seen nowadays, aluminum intoxication could be encountered with high content in the dialysis water source or with technical issues related to its treatment system [27, 28]. The resulting anemia is of microcytic hypochromic or normochromic pattern, which reflects ESA hyporesponsiveness associated with affected enzymes required for heme synthesis. Treatment requires gradual, incremental dosing of desferrioxamine infusion during hemodialysis sessions to avoid irreversible neurological damage. Other sources of aluminum exposure are aluminum-containing phosphate binders and antacids. The wide availability of-aluminum-containing phosphate binders led to very limited use of aluminum-containing phosphate binders for short periods and in certain occasions; for example, refractory hyperphosphatemia and hypercalcemia related to nonaluminum-containing phosphate binders. Combined use of sodium citrate with aluminum-containing phosphate binders promotes aluminum intoxication. Through increment of intestinal absorption. A concern was raised regarding the intake of ferric citrate as a phosphate binder due to the possible increase of aluminum absorption from food, water drinking, and concurrent medication use. Additional medications considered sources of aluminum are iron and calcium-containing medications, calcitriol vitamin B complex acetylsalicylic acid, clonidine, vitamins calcium carbonate, and iron sulfate. Injectable medications including iron, erythropoietin, and insulin have been found markedly more aluminum contaminated than oral formulations. Abnormal serum aluminum levels are those exceeding 20 mcg/L. According to Kidney Disease Outcomes Quality Initiative (KDOQI) guidelines, serum aluminum levels should be tested at least annually in hemodialysis patients and every 3 months in those who are taking aluminum-containing medications.

The Association for the Advancement of Medical Instrumentation (AAMI) recommendation is to perform periodic chemical monitoring for dialysis water at least annually, more frequently when indicated. The maximum allowed aluminum concentration is 0.01 mg/L [29–32].

4.5 Malnutrition

Protein-energy wasting and inflammation are closely associated. Malnutrition-inflammation complex is considered a predisposing factor for an impaired response to ESA therapy [33]. Moreover, vitamin deficiencies can be considered a contributing factor. Folic acid is involved in erythroid proliferation. Vitamin C, with its antioxidative effect, downregulates cytokine synthesis and increases iron utilization. Copper increases iron absorption. Alpha-lipoic acid is needed for ATP synthesis, and it has a lowering effect on symmetric-dimethyl arginine, reducing oxidative stress. L-Carnitine has an antioxidative stress effect by stimulating heme-oxygenase 1. There is no available data to support a relation between vitamin six and ESA hyporesponsiveness [34–37].

4.6 Pure red cell aplasia (PRCA)

As a consequence of epoetin-induced polyclonal antibodies, neutralization of exogenous ESA and cross-reaction with endogenous EPO occur [38]. So, erythropoiesis becomes defective with undetectable EPO levels in serum. The resulting rare condition is called pure red cell aplasia (PRCA). It is manifested by a rapid drop of Hb and undetectable reticulocytes with normal counts of white blood cells and platelets. PRCA is suspected with a monthly decrease of Hb level by 2 gm/dl or more r if reticulocyte count is less than 20,000/microL. It is usually thought of when hyporesponsiveness is preceded by a reasonable response to ESA therapy. For PRCA to occur, at least 3–4 weeks of EPO therapy must be there, with the typical presentation following 6–18 months of intake [39]. According to Kidney Disease Improving Global Outcomes (KDIGO) 012 guidelines, screening for PRCA due to anti-EPO antibodies in patients on EPO therapy for at least 4 weeks was suggested with absolute reticulocyte count less than 10,000/microL, normal platelet and white blood cell count, in addition, to drop of Hb level more than 0.5–1.0 g/dl weekly or need for 1–2 transfusions per week [40].

All PRCA cases induced by anti-EPO antibodies were reported after subcutaneous ESA administration, with a duration of treatment ranging from 1 month to 5 years [41]. PRCA mandates blood transfusion and immunosuppression, sometimes with rituximab [42]. Following the disappearance of EPO antibodies, IV ESA administration can be restarted with strict monitoring of anti-EPO antibody titers and Hb levels. Renal transplantation is the definitive solution.

4.7 Other causes

- CKD-mineral bone disease I interrelation among vitamin D, hyperparathyroidism, and hyporesponsive to ESA therapy is well known [43]. Vitamin D deficiency has a negative effect on erythropoiesis. Higher levels of parathyroid hormone inhibit erythroid progenitors and reduce red cell survival. Hyperphosphatemia leads to the downregulation of erythropoietin receptors. Hyperparathyroidism can be complicated by bone marrow fibrosis [44]. Higher levels of fibroblast growth factor-23 and alkaline phosphatase are considered biomarkers of ESA hyporesponssiveness [45].

- Angiotensin-converting enzyme inhibitors and angiotensin-receptor blockers: they inhibit angiotensin-II-induced EPO production and promote N-acetyl-seryl-aspartyl-lysyl-proline preventing recruitment of pluripotent stem cells; among other mechanisms [46].

- Bone marrow disorders: either primary or due to myelosuppressive agents.

- Malignancies: especially of hematological origin, for example, multiple myeloma and chronic lymphocytic leukemia [47].

- Hypothyroidism: higher TSH levels have been found to be related to decreased responsiveness to ESA therapy [48].

- Hypogonadism: the association has been found between lower testosterone levels and decreased response to ESA therapy [49].

- Hypomagnesemia: magnesium deficiency can increase oxidative stress and lead to the production of pro-inflammatory cytokines (TNF-alfa and IL-1B), decreasing ESA responsiveness. Serum magnesium levels were correlated with high ERI [50].

5. Suggested stepwise approach to ESA hyporesponsiveness

1. Step One: Exclude noncompliance to ESA therapy, especially in subcutaneous self-administration patients and those financial issues.

2. Step Two: Evaluate the proliferative status through estimation of reticulocyte count: Hyperproliferative state: we investigate for possible gastrointestinal bleeding using endoscopy or the possibility of hemolysis with testing of blood film, bilirubin, LDH, and Coombs test.

3. Step Three: Hypoproliferative state: We proceed for iron profile evaluation: Ferritin, TSAT, and HRC % to exclude functional and absolute iron deficiency.

4. Step Four: Hypoproliferative state; Exclusion of infection, inflammation, and inadequate dialysis: evaluation of kt/v CRP, together with a physical examination to exclude thrombosed arteriovenous graft, occult infection, failed kidney allograft, and infected dialysis access.

5. Step Five: Hypoproliferative state; Exclusion of vitamin deficiencies; Hb electrophoresis if indicated. Discontinuation of medications disturbing bone marrow erythropoiesis.

6. Step Six: Hypoproliferative state, Exclusion of hyperparathyroidism.

7. Step Seven: Undetectable reticulocytic count: Consideration of PRCA (**Figure 1**).

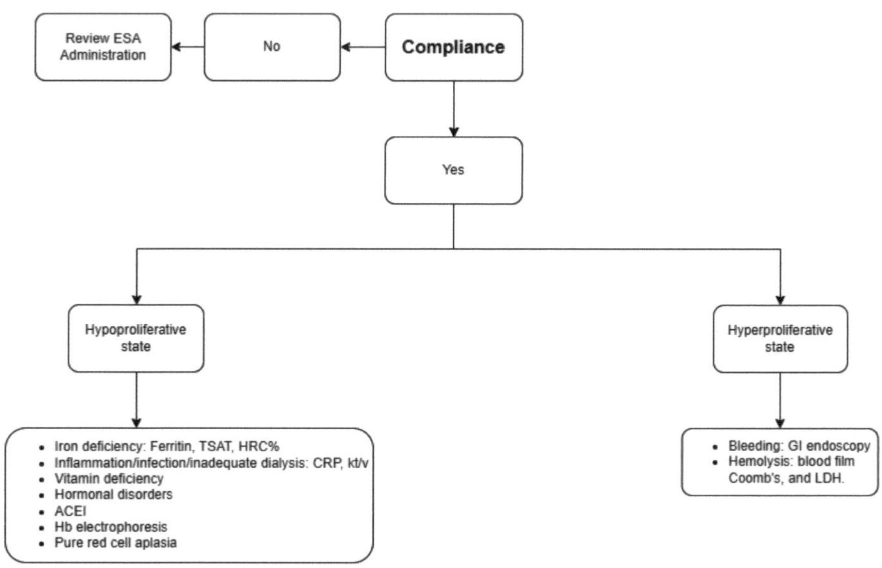

Figure 1.
Suggested stepwise approach to ESA hyporesponsiveness. TSAT: transferrin saturation, HRC%: hypochromic red blood cell %, CRP: C-reactive protein, GI: gastrointestinal, ACEI: angiotensin-converting enzyme inhibitor, and LDH: lactate dehydrogenase.

6. Clinical outcomes

Hyporesposiveness to ESA therapy has been found to be associated with higher mortality in several trials [51]. This was shown by one observational study of dialysis patients with Hb levels less than 9.5 gm/dl during larger ESA dose changes over 11 months period. The increased mortality has been in the initial period of therapy as shown by Trial to Reduce Cardiovascular Events with Aranesp Therapy (TREAT) study [52].

Both the underlying cause of ESA hyporesponsiveness and the ESA dose itself contributes to increased mortality, with the former having more importance [53]. ESA hyporesponsiveness has been associated with the development of insulin resistance [54]. Impaired response to ESA therapy can contribute through an unknown mechanism to more rapid progression to end-stage renal disease. This was suggested through a study of 194 consecutive CKD patients on ESA therapy between 2002 and 2006 [55].

7. Potential and investigational agents

7.1 Hypoxia-inducible factor-prolyl hydroxylase inhibitors (HIF-PHIs)

Also, they are called HIF stabilizers. The major transcription factor for the EPO gene, HIF, was discovered in 1992. This was followed by the creation of HIF stabilizers. Their action process is via the HIF-prolyl hydroxylase domain (PHD) pathway through stimulation of transcription of EPO gene resulting in increased endogenous EPO levels. Anemia-induced tissue hypoxia leads to HIF system stimulation. Intranuclear dislocation of HIF-alpha is followed by its binding to HIF-B to form a functional dimer that binds to hypoxia-response elements on DNA. Eventually, HIF induces the expression of genes regulating erythropoiesis and iron metabolism in a wide range of tissues. HIF activity and degradation are regulated by PHD proteins. They are oxygen-sensitive hydroxylase enzymes. Their activity decreases during conditions of hypoxia. Development of CKD leads to HIF dysregulation with reduced EPO production. HIF-PHIs enhance the physiologic response to hypoxia through suppression of PHD leading to endogenous EPO production with Hb overshoots less than ESA therapy. HIF-PHIs have direct and indirect beneficial effects on iron deficiency, either absolute or functional type. Directly, HIF-PHIs regulate iron homeostasis proteins, for example, duodenal cytochrome B, ferroportin, transferrin, and divalent metal-ion transporter 1. Indirectly, HIF-PHIs have suppression action on hepcidin (via erythroferrone, the main hepcidin-erythroid regulator), leading to a possible increase in iron availability [56, 57].

Agents of this novel class included in clinical trials are: daprodustat, vadadustat, and raxadustat; all are used orally.

The safety and efficacy of the HIF PHI daprodustat were evaluated in a trial of 2964 patients on dialysis over 2.5 years (average hemoglobin 10.4 g/L) who were randomly given daprodustat (dose range from 4 to 24 mg daily, according to ESA dose) or injectable ESA (epoetin alfa hemodialysis patients or darbepoetin alfa for peritoneal dialysis patients). The average change in Hb concentration was 0.28 g/dL with daprodustat therapy and 0.10 g/dL with ESA therapy. Rates of adverse cardiovascular events, a composite of death, nonfatal myocardial infarction, and stroke, were similar between the treatment groups (25.2 versus 26.7% for daprodustat and epoetin alfa, respectively), as were the rates of other adverse events. The efficacy of another dosing of daprodustat was studied in a 52-week trial in which 407 patients on hemodialysis were randomly assigned to daprodustat (dose range from 2 to 48 mg) thrice weekly with dialysis or to epoetin alfa; the average change in Hb concentration and rates of adverse events were similar between the treatment groups.

The efficacy and safety of vadadustat have been studied in comparison to Darbepoetin alfa in hemodialysis patients in a trial of 3554 patients who were randomly assigned to receive vadadustat 150–600 mg or darbepoetin alfa. to target Hb of 10 to 11 g/dL in patients of the United States and 10 to 12 g/dL in patients from other countries. Iron was given to all participants targeting transferrin saturation (TSAT) >20 percent and serum ferritin >100 ng/mL. Between weeks 40 and 52, prevalent dialysis patients assigned to vadadustat were less likely to maintain target Hb (44 versus 51 percent), although rates of red cell transfusion were similar (2.0 vs. 1.9% of prevalent dialysis patients). Findings from a similar trial of 369 incident patients on dialysis showed comparable results.

Collectively, data of patients from both trials, rates of mortality (13.0 vs. 12.9%, nonfatal stroke (1.3 vs. 1.9%), hospitalization for heart failure (3.9 vs. 4.0%), and nonfatal myocardial infarction (3.9 vs. 4.5%) were comparable. Other adverse events, for example, hypertension, diarrhea, and pneumonia, were lower in the vadadustat group; both among prevalent (55 vs. 58%) and incident (50 vs. 57%) dialysis patients [58, 59].

Similar findings have been obtained from smaller studies of roxadustat in comparison to findings of studies of daprodustat and vadadustat [60].

As roxadustat is a selective activity ligand for thyroid hormone receptor B; with its similar structure to T3, it can suppress TSH release.

These agents have gained acceptance for clinical use in Europe, China, Japan, and Chile but not yet in the United States.

Long-term follow-up is required for concerns like increased risk of cancer, cardiovascular events, thrombosis, and deterioration of diabetic retinopathy, among others [61–63].

7.2 Experimental combination of ESA and thrombopoietin

The use of ESA and thrombopoietin in combination to treat EPO-resistant anemia in otherwise healthy rats was suggested based on the ability of thrombopoietin to stimulate self-renewal of stem cells and correct depletion of erythroid precursor cells [64].

7.3 L-carnitine

Dialysis patients are in a state of chronic carnitine deficiency, associated with fatty acid and other organic acid metabolic disturbances. Observational studies showed a relation between elevated ERI and low L-carnitine. However, other studies did not show evidence of beneficial effects regarding oxidative stress and inflammation in hemodialysis patients [65].

7.4 Pentoxifylline

It has anti-inflammatory effects through inhibition of the production of TNF-alpha and IFN-gamma. This was shown with oral pentoxifylline given to dialysis patients hyporesponsive to ESA therapy with a resulting significant improvement of Hb levels in a small open-label study. However, CRP levels were not changed. Further studies did not support the clinical utility of pentoxifylline in anemic dialysis patients [66].

7.5 AST-120

It is an inert binding compound with an antioxidant effect and the capability to reduce uremic toxins, indoxyl sulfate, and p-cresyl sulfate levels. Some improvement of anemia was shown in a crossover study with AST-120 given to predialysis patients [67].

7.6 Vitamin E-coated dialyzer

There is controversy regarding its effects on oxidative stress, inflammation, and ESA responsiveness. However, direct relation was suggested between the higher positive effect of vitamin E-coated dialyzer and higher levels of ERI [68].

7.7 Anti-hepcidin agents

Lexaptepid pegol and human anti-BMP6 antibodies are hepcidin-suppressing agents. Experimental use of anti-BMP6 antibodies reduced the need for EPO in the treatment of anemia of chronic disease. Other agents targeting the ferroportin degradation action of hepcidin are for underway research [69].

7.8 Alpha-lipoic acid

In a multicenter prospective randomized study, it was shown that alpha-lipoic acid in a dose of 600 mg/day had anti-inflammatory and antioxidant effects leading to improvement of anemia and EPO resistance in diabetic patients on hemodialysis. Further studies are required for complete evaluation with the use of different doses [70].

7.9 Statin therapy

In a meta-analysis study, it was found that CKD patients treated with a statin had a trend of increased Hb and decreased ferritin levels. Further studies are required for more result validation [71].

7.10 SGLT2 inhibitors

They have been shown to have a beneficial effect on anemia reduction through decreasing hepcidin and ferritin and increasing transferrin [72].

8. Conclusion

Hyporesponse to ESA therapy has well-known negative outcomes in hemodialysis patients. A wise approach is to target the underlying causes before the up-titration of the ESA dose. There is insufficient evidence of adjuvant therapy and adverse effects of exogenous ESA as well. The discovery of new areas of hepcidin and HIF pathway paved the way for the possible development of novel therapeutic agents, including EPO gene therapy, hepcidin antagonists, and better-planned tackling HIF stabilizers. More dedicated efforts are still required for better-planned tackling of a problem that has continued for more than two decades.

Acknowledgements

For the technical support, we would like to thank Ahmed Mahrous, Pharmacy Department, Ashmoun Health Center, Monofiya, Egypt.

Funding sources

There was no external funding for this work.

Conflict of interest

The authors have no conflicts of interest to declare.

Author details

Ahmed Yasin[1*] and Nayer Omran[2]

1 Nephrology Division, Internal Medicine Department, Saudi German Hospital, Medina, Saudi Arabia

2 School of Medicine, New Giza University, Giza, Egypt

*Address all correspondence to: nephrology20192019@gmail.com

References

[1] Cappellini MD et al. Anemia in clinical practice-definition and classification: Does hemoglobin change with aging? Seminars in Hematology. Oct 2015;**52**(4):261-269

[2] Locatelli F, Pisoni RL, Combe C, Bommer J, Andreucci VE, Piera L, et al. Anaemia in haemodialysis patients of five European countries: Association with morbidity and mortality in the Dialysis outcomes and practice patterns study (DOPPS). Nephrology, Dialysis, Transplantation. 2004;**19**(1):121-132

[3] Taddei S, Nami R, Bruno RM, Quatrini I, Nuti R. Hypertension left ventricular hypertrophy and chronic kidney disease. Heart Failure Review. 2011;**16**(6):615-620

[4] Babitt JL, Lin HY. Mechanisms of anemia in CKD. Journal of American Society Nephrology. 2012;**23**(10):1631-1634

[5] Bahlmann FH, Kielstein JT, Haller H, Fliser D. Erythropoietin and progression of CKD. Kidney International. 2007;**107**:S21-S25

[6] Batchelor EK, Kapitsinou P, Pergola PE, Kovesdy CP, Jalal DI. Iron deficiency in chronic kidney disease: Updates on pathophysiology, diagnosis, and treatment. Journal of American Society Nephrology. 2020;**31**(3):456-468

[7] Eschbach JW, Abdulhadi MH, Browne JK, Delano BG, Downing MR, Egrie JC, et al. Recombinant human erythropoietin in anemic patients with end-stage renal disease. Results of a phase III multicenter clinical trial. Annals of Internal Medicine. 1989;**111**:992

[8] Luo J, Jensen DE, Maroni BJ, Brunelli SM. Spectrum and burden erythropoiesis-stimulating agent hyporesponsiveness among contemporary hemodialysis patients. American Journal of Kidney Diseases. 2016;**86**:763

[9] Sibbel SP, Koro CE, Brunelli SM, Cobitz AR. Characterization of chronic and acute ESA hyporesponse: A retrospective cohort study of hemodialysis patients. BMC Nephrology. 2015;**16**:144

[10] Locatelli F, Aljama P, Bárány P, et al. Revised European best practice guidelines for the management of anaemia in patients with chronic renal failure. Nephrology, Dialysis, Transplantation. 2004;**19**:ii1

[11] Chapter 1: Diagnosis and evaluation of anemia in CKD. Kidney International Supplements. 2011;**2012**(2):288

[12] Chait Y et al. The greatly misunderstood erythropoietin resistance index and the case for a new responsiveness measure. Hemodialysis International. 2016;**20**(3):392-398

[13] Gilbertson DT et al. Comparison of methodologies to define hemodialysis patients hypo-responsive to epoetin and impact on counts and characteristics. BMC Nephrology. 2013;**14**:44

[14] Drueke T. Hyporesponsiveness to recombinant human erythropoietin. Nephrology, Dialysis, Transplantation. 2001;**16**(suppl):725-728

[15] Laura E et al. Diagnosis and management of iron deficiency in CKD: A summary of the NICE guideline recommendations and their rationale. American Journal of Kidney Diseases. Apr 2016;**67**(4):548-558

[16] Madu AJ, Ughansoro MD. Anemia of chronic disease: An in-depth review. Medical Principles and Practice. 2017;**26**(1):1-9

[17] Goicoechea M, Martin J, de Sequera P, et al. Role of cytokines in the response to erythropoietin in hemodialysis patients. Kidney International. 1998;**54**:1337

[18] Nassar GM, Fishbane S, Ayus JC. Occult infection of old nonfunctioning arteriovenous grafts: A novel cause of erythropoietin resistance and chronic inflammation in hemodialysis patients. Kidney International Supplement. May 2002;(80):49-54

[19] Solid CA, Foley RN, Gill JS, et al. Epoetin use and kidney disease outcomes quality initiative hemoglobin targets in patients returning to dialysis with failed renal transplants. Kidney International. 2007;**71**:425

[20] Movilli E, Cancarini GC, Zani R, et al. Adequacy of dialysis reduces the doses of recombinant erythropoietin independently from the use of biocompatible membranes in haemodialysis patients. Nephrology, Dialysis, Transplantation. 2001;**16**:111

[21] Locatelli F, Del Vecchio L. Dialysis adequacy and response to erythropoietic agents: What is the evidence base? Nephrology, Dialysis, Transplantation. 2003;**18**(Suppl 8):viii29

[22] Hsu PY, Lin CL, Yu CC, et al. Ultrapure dialysate improves iron utilization and erythropoietin response in chronic hemodialysis patients—A prospective cross-over study. Journal of Nephrology. 2004;**17**:693

[23] Yang J et al. Efficacy of medium cut-off dialyzer and comparison with high-flux dialyzers in patients on maintenance hemodialysis: A systematic review and q meta-analysis. Therapeutic Apheresis and Dialysis. Aug 2002;**26**(4):756-768

[24] Yaqoob MM et al. Resistance to recombinant human erythropoietin due to aluminium overload and its removal by low dose desferrioxamine therapy. Postgraduate Medical Journal. 1993;**69**(808):124

[25] Bohrer D et al. Role of medication in the level of aluminium in the blood of chronic hemodialysis patients. Nephrology Dialysis Transplantation. 2009;**24**(4):1277-1281

[26] Zhao Y et al. Efficacy and safety of expanded hemodialysis patients: A meta-analysis and systematic review. Renal Failure. 2022;**44**(1):541-550

[27] Zhang Z. Effects of expanded hemodialysis with medium cut-off membranes on maintenance hemodialysis patients: A review. Membranes. 2022;**12**:253

[28] Jofre R et al. Inflammatory syndrome in patients on hemodialysis. Journal of American Society of Nephrology. 2006;**17**(12):S274-S280

[29] Bamonti-Catena F et al. Folate measurement in patients on regular hemodialysis treatment. American Journal of Kidney Diseases. 1999;**33**(3):492-497

[30] Bridges KR, Hoffman KE. The effects of ascorbic acid on the intracellular metabolism of iron and ferritin. The Journal of Biological Chemistry. 1986;**261**(30):14273-14277

[31] Tan BL et al. Nutrients and oxidative stress: Friend or foe? The Journal of Biological Chemistry, Oxidative Medical Cell Longevity. 2018;**2018**:719584

[32] Froment DP, Molitoris BA, Buddington B, et al. Site and mechanism of enhanced gastrointestinal absorption of aluminum by citrate. Kidney International. 1989;**36**:978

[33] Van Buren PN, Lewis JB, Dwyer JP, et al. The phosphate binder ferric citrate and mineral metabolism and inflammatory markers in maintenance Dialysis patients: Results from Prespecified analyses of a randomized clinical trial. American Journal of Kidney Diseases. 2015;**66**:479

[34] Gupta A. Ferric citrate hydrate as a phosphate binder and risk of aluminum toxicity. Pharmaceuticals (Basel). 2014;**7**:990

[35] Bohrer D, Bertagnolli DC, de Oliveira SM, et al. Drugs as a hidden source of aluminium for chronic renal patients. Nephrology, Dialysis, Transplantation. 2007;**22**:605

[36] Association for the Advancement of Medical instrumentation(AAMI) Standards, Dialysis, 2013 Edition

[37] Calo LA et al. Carnitine-mediated improved response to erythropoietin involves induction of heme oxygenase-1: Studies in humans and in animal model. Nephrology, Dialysis, Transplantation. 2008;**23**(3):890-895

[38] Casadevall N, Nataf J, Viron B, et al. Pure red-cell aplasia and antierythropoietin antibodies in patients treated with recombinant erythropoietin. The New England Journal of Medicine. 2002;**346**:469

[39] Rossert J, Casadevall N, Eckardt KU. Anti-erythropoietin antibodies and pure red cell aplasia. Journal of American Society Nephrology. 2004;**15**:398

[40] Quint L, Casadevall N, Giraudiet S. Pure red cell aplasia in patients ith refractory anemia treated with two different recombinant erythropoietins. British Journal of Hematology. 2004;**124**:842

[41] Verhelst D et al. Treatment of erythropoietin -induced pure red cell aplasia: A retrospective study. Lancet. 2004;**363**:1768

[42] Bamgbola OF. Pattern of resistance to erythropoietin-stimulating agents in chronic kidney disease. Kidney International. 2011;**80**(5):464-474

[43] Del Vecchio L et al. Inflammation and resistance to treatment with recombinant human erythropoiesis. Renal Nutrition. 2005;**15**(1):137-141

[44] Usui T et al. Association of erythropoietin resistance and fibroblast growth factor 23 in dialysis patients: Results from the Japanese dialysis outcomes and practice patterns study. Nephrology. 2021;**26**(1):46-53

[45] Aiz M et al. Acute angiotensin-converting enzyme inhibition increases the plasma levels of the natural stem cell regulator N-acetyl-seryl-aspartyl-lysyl-proline. The Journal of Clinical Investigation. 1996;**97**(3):839-844

[46] Latcha S. Anemia management in cancer patients with chronic kidney disease. Seminars in Dialysis. 2019;**23**(6):513-519

[47] Saleh F et al. Effect of thyroid function status in hemodialysis patients on erythropoietin resistance and interdialytic weight gain. Kidney Diseases Transplantation. Nov-Dec 2018;**29**(6):1274-1279

[48] Stenvinkel P, Barany P. Hypogonadism in males with chronic kidney disease: another cause of resistance to erythropoiesis-stimulating

agents? Contributions to Nephrology. 2012;**178**:35-39

[49] Yu L et al. Association between serum magnesium and erythropoietin responsiveness in hemodialysis patients: A cross-sectional study. Kidney & Blood Pressure Research. 2019;**44**:354-361

[50] Bradbury BD et al. Effect of epoetin alfa dose changes on hemoglobin and mortality in hemodialysis patients with hemoglobin levels persistently below 11 gldL. Clinical American Society Nephrology. 2009;**4**:630

[51] Solomon SD et al. Erythropoietic response and outcomes in kidney disease and type 2 diabetes. The New England Journal of Medicine. 2010;**363**:1146

[52] Szczech LA et al. Secondary analysis of the CHOIR trial epoetin alfa dose and achieved hemoglobin outcomes. Kidney International. 2008;**74**:791

[53] Abe M et al. Relationship between insulin resistance and epoetin response in hemodialysis patients. Clinical Nephrology. Jan 2011;**75**(1):49-58

[54] Minutolo R et al. Hyporesponsiveness to erythropoiesis stimulating agents and renal survival in non-dialysis CKD patients. Nephrology, Dialysis, Transplantation. 2012;**27**:2880

[55] Nair Sand Trivedi M. Anemia management in dialysis patients: A PIVOT and a new path? Current Opinion in Nephrology Hypertension. 2020;**29**(3):351-355

[56] Rosenberger C et al. Expression of hypoxia-inducible factor-1 alfa and 2 alfa in hypoxic and ischemic rat kidneys. Journal of American Society of Nephrology. 2002;**13**(7):1721-1732

[57] Singh AK et al. Daprodustat for the treatment of anemia in patients undergoing dialysis. New England Journal of Medicine. 2021;**385**(25):2325

[58] Echardt KU et al. Safety and efficacy of Vadadustat for anemia in patients undergoing dialysis. New England Journal of Medicine. 2021;**384**(17):1601

[59] Liu Z et al. Roxadustat (FG-4592) treatment for anemia in dialysis-dependent (DD) and not dialysis-dependent (NDD) chronic kidney disease patients: A systematic review and meta-analysis. Pharmacological Research. 2020;**155**:104747

[60] Tokuyama A et al. Roxadustat and thyroid stimulating hormone suppression. Clinical Journal. 2021;**14**(5):1472-1474

[61] Yap DY et al. Recommendation by the Asian pacific society of nephrology 9APSN on the appropriate use of HIF-PH inhibitors. Nephrology. 2021;**26**(2):105-118

[62] Sanghani NS, Haase VH. Hypoxia-inducible factor activators in renal anemia : Current clinical experience. Advances in Chronic Kidney Disease. 2019;**26**(4):523

[63] Kular D, Macdougall I. HIF stabilizers in the management of renal anemia: From bench to bedside to pediatrics. Pediatric Nephrology. 2019;**34**:365-378

[64] Zou H. et al, A novel combination therapy of epoetin and thrombopoietin to treat epoetin-resistant anemia. Pharmaceutical Research. 2022;**39**:1249-1268

[65] Yang SK, Xiao L, Song PA, Xu X, Liu FY, Sun L. Effect of L-carnitine therapy on patients in maintenance hemodialysis: A systematic review and

meta-analysis. Journal of Nephrology. 2014;**27**(3):317-329

[66] Johnson DW, Pascoe EM, Badve SV, et al. A randomized, placebo-controlled trial of pentoxifylline on erythropoiesis-stimulating agent hypo-responsiveness in anemic patients with CKD: The handling erythropoietin resistance with Oxpentifylline (HERO) trial. American Journal of Kidney Diseases. 2015;**65**(1):49-57

[67] Wu IW, Hsu KH, Sun CY, Tsai CJ, Wu MS, Lee CC. Oral adsorbent AST-120 potentiates the effect of erythropoietin-stimulating agents on stage 5 chronic kidney disease patients: A randomizes crossover study. Nephrological Dialysis Transplantation. 2014;**29**(9):1719-1727

[68] Panichi V, Rosati A, Paoletti S, et al. A vitamin E-coated polysulfone membrane reduces serum levels of inflammatory markers and resistance to erythropoietin-stimulating agents in hemodialysis patients: Results of a randomized cross-over multicenter trial. Blood Purification. 2011;**32**:7-14

[69] Malyszko J, Malyszko JS, Matuszkiewics-Rowinska J. Hepcidin as a therapeutic target for anemia and inflammation associated with chronic kidney disease. Expert Opinion on Therapeutic Targets. 2019;**23**(5):407-421

[70] Abdel Hamid DZ et al. Alpha-lipoic acid improved anemia, erythropoietin resistance, maintained glycemic control, and reduced cardiovascular risk in diabetic patients on hemodialysis: A multicenter prospective randomized controlled study. European Review in Medicine & Pharmacological Science. 2022;**26**:2313-2329

[71] Tsai MH et al. The effect of statin on Anemia in patients with chronic kidney disease and end-stage kidney disease: A systematic review and Meta-analysis. Journal of Persian Medicine. 2022;**12**:1175

[72] Schmidt DW, Argyropoulos C, Sing N. Are the protective effects of SGLT2 inhibitors a 'class effect' or are there differences between agents? Kidney. 2021;**2**:881-885

Chapter 8

Psychosocial Aspects in Hemodialysis

Hayfa Almutary

Abstract

Several psychosocial stressors have an impact on patients with end-stage kidney disease (ESKD). The disease and its treatment modalities impose several lifestyle changes. These include the impact of disease and treatment, dietary and fluid restrictions, functional limitations and sexual dysfunction, and future uncertainty and fear of death. Furthermore, family and social issues such as changes in family roles and changes in duties and responsibilities may add to psychosocial stressors among people on dialysis. Commonly associated psychosocial issues include depression, anxiety, delirium, withdrawal, and decreased quality of life. The prevalence and severity of each psychological issue vary, and there are several tools available to detect these issues. This chapter will focus on the most common psychosocial stressors among people with hemodialysis.

Keywords: anxiety, depression, delirium, hemodialysis, psychosocial issue, stressors, withdrawal

1. Introduction

Over the past three decades, significant advancements in the knowledge of and understanding of the treatment of end-stage kidney disease (ESKD) have been made. According to the biopsychosocial model, which is linked to ESKD, dialysis has biological, psychological, and social consequences [1]. However, many studies focus on the biological effects of dialysis, and little attention has been given to psychosocial issues in hemodialysis. The psychosocial stressors that patients undergoing dialysis therapy face are numerous. Based on the psychosocial model, each person is unique, and his or her stressors interact with each other, which illustrates their complexity [1].

Several psychosocial stressors have an impact on patients with ESKD. The disease and its treatment modalities impose several lifestyle changes. These include the impact of disease and treatment, dietary and fluid restrictions, functional limitations and sexual dysfunction, and future uncertainty and fear of death. Furthermore, family and social issues such as changes in family roles and changes in duties and responsibilities may add to psychosocial stressors among people on dialysis. Some of these stressors among dialysis patients may cause changes in patients' marital and occupational status, which lead to isolation and decrease quality of life. Commonly associated psychosocial issues include depression, anxiety, delirium, and withdrawal from dialysis. These stressors may differ in their occurrence and manifestation according to the time of the dialysis. Understanding these issues and their impact on patients undergoing dialysis therapy will have positive implications for clinical practice and patients' outcomes. Priority should be given to prevention and early identification of these issues throughout the trajectory of the dialysis treatment. This chapter will focus on the most common psychosocial issues among people on hemodialysis.

2. Psychosocial issues in the transition to hemodialysis

The actual transition from chronic renal care to hemodialysis therapy results in a new challenge for patients' lives across all aspects [2]. This transition period is critical and associated with many psychological stressors. Future uncertainty, being a burden on family, financial strain, transportation issues, physical dysfunction, lifestyle and schedule changes, and travel restrictions are all sources of psychological stressors. In fact, many patients experience shock when they are told to start dialysis [3]. This initial shock event can lead to a serious psychological crisis. The patient may experience denial, regret, depression, anxiety, worry, anger, sleep disturbances, grief, and isolation [4]. Moreover, newly commenced dialysis patients may experience identity alterations because of altered body image, dependence, frailty, and loss of identity [5]. During the initial hemodialysis, patients often deny the fact that dialysis has become part of their lives and is a permanent treatment [6]. Denial is regarded as a protective mechanism for dealing with emotional stressors associated with dialysis [7]. Denial may lead to a refusal to adhere to dietary and fluid restrictions and a testing of what happens when they break boundaries. In some cases, this may lead to withdrawal or decreased compliance with dialysis [7]. A previous study reported a correlation between withdrawal and early dialysis initiation [8]. The first year on hemodialysis is a central period for adaptation and coping [5]. Perhaps it is only a matter of time before the patient accepts the fact that dialysis is sustaining their life. Indeed, when patients' health deteriorated significantly, they eventually accepted the reality of dialysis and followed the instructions.

In a qualitative study that explored patient experience after the first year of dialysis, family and dialysis acceptance and coping were the dominant psychosocial stressors [2, 5]. Patients feel that hemodialysis affects social interaction and changes their relationships. Furthermore, physical and psychosocial functions affect their ability to work and be independent. Studies show that the first years of initiating hemodialysis are associated with changes in employment status and reduce the income [9, 10]. Given this, depression and social isolation may become apparent until the patient accepts and adapts to the new treatment [5].

Transitioning from other treatment modalities, such as peritoneal dialysis, to hemodialysis is required in some cases. This transition also imposes some psychological issues [11]. Patients are frequently hesitant to accept or change a treatment at first [11]. These patients may also experience similar psychological issues (e.g., depression, fear, and anxiety) as patients who have been transferred from pre-dialysis care to hemodialysis for the first time.

2.1 Psychosocial care in the initial period of hemodialysis

Assessment of psychological status should be an integral part of hemodialysis care, especially during the transition period. To facilitate a healthy transition to hemodialysis, clinicians should be alert during this critical period for any changes in emotion and mood and provide social and emotional support [2]. A patient-centered approach of care should be applied through individual evaluation of each patient to meet his or her supporting needs. It is critical to provide effective training and educational programs for patients and their families in order to improve acceptance and coping with hemodialysis. Moreover, providing opportunity to share experience and talking to other patients on dialysis will help in this regard.

New patients may be reluctant to ask questions or express their feelings. Establishing a trust relationship between patients and healthcare professionals improves the patient experience and facilitates coping mechanisms [5]. This relationship will enable information sharing, promote self-efficacy and management, support decision-making, and reduce depression and anxiety.

3. Depression

Depression is a common mental disorder worldwide. According to the American Psychiatric Association, depression is a common illness that negatively affects feelings, thinking, and responses [12]. It is an emotional state marked by somatic and cognitive symptoms [13]. Depression is often known as major depressive disorder or clinical depression, which is widely underreported and underdiagnosed in many chronic illnesses.

The National institute of Mental Health indicates that depression has various types [14]. These are major depression, persistent depressive disorder, perinatal depression, seasonal affective disorder, and depression with symptoms of psychosis. The major depression is defined by symptoms that last at least 2 weeks and interfere with daily activities. More specifically, the Diagnostic and Statistical Manual for Mental Disorders (DSM-5) in its latest version indicates that the diagnosis of a major depressive disorder should have two criteria. First, the symptoms should continue for a period of at least 2 weeks. Second, depressed mood should be experienced almost daily or be accompanied by a loss of interest in routine activities, as well as at least four of the additional symptoms listed below: (a) significant change in weight (either loss or gain) or change in appetite, (b) alteration in sleep pattern (e.g., insomnia), (c) psychomotor changes (i.e., agitation or retardation), (d) fatigue and loss of energy, (e) feelings of worthlessness or extreme guilt, (f) decreased concentration, or (g) thoughts of death or suicide [15] Cohen et al. noted that many of these symptoms that are associated with major depression could overlap with uremic symptoms in ESKD [16]. However, death and suicidal thoughts are more likely to be related to major depression. It is therefore important that clinicians be careful when they assess depression in this specific population.

The other type of depression is persistent depressive disorder, which is also called dysthymia, and is characterized by a lower severity of the depressive symptoms but a longer duration, typically at least 2 years. Perinatal depression is experienced by women and associated with specific times such as pregnancy and the postpartum period. Seasonal affective disorder has been linked to particular seasons. The last type is depression with symptoms of psychosis, which is the most severe type of depression in which psychosis symptoms also occur.

Depression in hemodialysis is contributed by numerous changes in the personal, social, and professional aspects, such as job loss, dietary changes, and sexual dysfunction, in addition to the frequent stressful experience of dialysis, the invasive procedure of dialysis, issues related to dialysis access, uncertainty about the future, and anxiety regarding mortality. The adverse outcomes of depression among hemodialysis have been widely examined. Previous studies indicate that depression among dialysis patients is associated with poor treatment adherence [17, 18], high hospitalization rates [19], and lower quality of life [20, 21]. There is growing evidence that the depression is correlated with increased risk of mortality rates in hemodialysis [19, 21–24]. Cheng et al. found that cognitive symptoms of depression have a better predictive value of long-term mortality in people undergoing hemodialysis than somatic symptoms [25]. Collectively, the adverse effects of depression make it an important subject to address.

Globally, depression affects approximately 5% of adults and is the principal cause of disability [26]. Moreover, it is one of the most common mental disorders among hemodialysis patients. The prevalence of depression varies among countries. However, a large body of literature shows that depression affects about one-quarter of dialysis patients [27–29]. In the USA, the prevalence of depression among hemodialysis patients ranges between 14 and 44% [30, 31], and in Australia, it was found to be about 13.3% [32]. A multinational European study conducted in Portugal, Turkey, Italy, and France that examined depression among 2278 people with hemodialysis reported a prevalence as 46% [33]. Depression rates in Saudi Arabia ranged from 5.62% to 44.7% [34, 35]. Depression in hemodialysis was much higher in Africa, as it ranged between 45 and 76.3% [36]. The variation across these studies was due to the potential for variation in methodological designs applied and assessment measures utilized, in addition to other factors such as sex, race, educational level, and economic status.

3.1 Screening and diagnostic measures

There are several measures available to diagnose and screen for depression in hemodialysis units. The semistructured interviews are considered the gold-standard method of diagnosis for depression. These include the Mini International Neuropsychiatric Interview and the Structured Clinical Interview for DSM-IV Axis I Disorders (SCID-1) [37]. These types of interviews should be conducted by well-skilled healthcare professionals who are familiar with the criteria for the diagnosis of major depression mentioned previously.

Given the dramatic changes in all aspects of life for people undergoing hemodialysis, it is recommended to screen for depression at the time of initiation, after 6 months, and then yearly [38]. It is also supported by prior evidence demonstrating that there is no correlation between any specific time since the commencement of dialysis and the occurrence of depression [39]. This requires ongoing examination of depression in hemodialysis patients throughout their treatment trajectory. Currently, the Beck Depression Inventory, Patient Health Questionnaire (PHQ-9), Center for Epidemiologic Studies Depression Scale (CES-D), and Hospital Anxiety and Depression Scale (HADS) are valid and reliable measures for screening of depression the dialysis population. Although the best one to use remains uncertain. These measures differ in their lengths and items, which make some of them more efficient for initial screening of depression.

The most commonly used measure to assess depression is the Beck Depression Inventory (BDI). It has been extensively used in screening patients with ESKD [40]. The BDI was developed in 1961 and consisted of 21 items [41]. Over time, the scale has been revised to be updated according to the new guidelines and diagnostic criteria for psychological disorders issued by the American Psychiatric Association. The first version of BDI (BDI-I) was published in 1987. Then, the second version of BDI (BDI-II) was available in 1996 and included 21 items as well as a few items revised [41]. This scale evaluates responses on a 4-point Likert scale, where 0 means that no problem exists and 3 means that the problem is highly prevalent. The maximum score of the BDI-II is 63. The severity of the depression was classified based on the range of scores given. When the BDI-II score ranges from 0 to 13, it is considered minimal depression. When the score is between 14 and 19, it indicates mild depression. When a person's BDI-II score ranges from 20 to 28, they may be suffering from moderate depression. Severe depression is classified when the BDI-II score ranges from 29 to 63 [42]. In addition, a cutoff score of ≥11 was identified as sensitive point for determining the major depressive episode among patients with chronic kidney disease [43]. The BDI-II is a well-validated scale that has been used widely used to assess depression in people undergoing dialysis [44–49].

The latest version of BDI is known as BDI-FS, which is fast and short and includes only seven items. The scale of scoring is 0–3. The value of this version is to accelerate the screening for depression. This quick scale may be useful in identifying potential hemodialysis patients who are depressed [36, 50], and once identified, further testing should be performed to validate the diagnosis and initiate the appropriate intervention.

It was argued that developing a tool that focuses on non-somatic disturbances associated with depression while excluding somatic symptoms that could be caused by dialysis is critical. Accordingly, the Cognitive Depression Index (CDI) was developed by selecting a subset of 15 items from the BDI-II and excluding those related to somatic symptoms [37, 51]. The significance of this index was emphasized by both Kimmel et al. and Peterson et al., who found a correlation between high depression using CDI and increased mortality rates and lower survival rates in chronic kidney disease [52, 53].

Additional short and fast tool for screening of depression is the Patient Health Questionnaire (PHQ-9). It is a self-reported survey that includes nine items specific to depression. The responses are scored on a 4-point scale to indicate the severity of depression, with 0 for a statement indicating not at all and 3 indicating experience with a statement of nearly every day. A maximum score assumed for the PHQ-9 is 27. Using this measure, depression is classified into four categories. A score range between 1 and 4 indicates that there is no depression, a score range between 5 and 9 indicates a mild depression, a score range between 10 and 14 indicates a moderate depression, a score range between 15 and 19 indicates a moderately severe depression, and a score of 20 or more indicates a severe depression [54]. A previous study suggested that a cutoff point of 10 on the PHQ-9 is sensitive to detecting depressed patients [55]. As the PHQ-9 is also short, it is recommended to use it as a screening tool for depression in dialysis units.

Another well-known measure for assessing depression in hemodialysis is the Hospital Anxiety and Depression Scale (HADS). It was developed in 1983 by Zigmond and Snaith to evaluate both anxiety and depression levels in the outpatient units of the hospital [56]. HADS is a relatively short and quick instrument. It is a self-reported survey with 14 multiple-choice questions that have two subscales: anxiety (HADS-A) and depression (HADS-D). Each subscale includes seven items rated on a four-point scale (from 0 to 3), where 0 indicates the absence of the problem and 3 indicates the presence and severity of the problem. The maximum score given is 21. A score of 7 or less means absence of anxiety or depression; a score between 8 and 10 represents moderate levels of anxiety or depression; and score more than 11 reveals high levels of anxiety or depression. The HADS is a valid tool, and extensive studies show that HADS is practical in the assessment of anxiety and depression among people undergoing hemodialysis [57–61].

Center for Epidemiologic Studies Depression Scale (CES-D) is one of the most common instruments used to assess depression. The Center for Epidemiological Studies-Depression (CES-D) created this scale to assess depression in 1977 by Radloff [62]. It comprises 20 items that evaluate the mood and somatic symptoms, interpersonal relationships, and motor functioning in the past week. The total score of the scale ranges from 0 to 60, with a higher score revealing worse psychological status. A cutoff value of ≥16 was approved to indicate depression. The scale was validated and used in many studies for patient undergoing hemodialysis [37, 63]. Other screening measures have been used to assess depression among hemodialysis patients using non-specific tools and parts of other tools, such as the Kidney Disease Quality of Life Questionnaire (KDQOL-SF), the SF-36, the Mental Health Inventory 5, and the Edmonton Symptom Assessment System.

It is important to notice that using self-reporting scales could result in overdiagnosis, especially among patients on dialysis. The daily symptoms experienced by those patients (e.g., fatigue, sleep disturbance, and difficult concentration) can overlap with the somatic symptoms of depression. Besides the symptom burden, the occurrence of other comorbid conditions may add to the complexity of the depression diagnosis in a patient on dialysis.

3.2 Management of depression in hemodialysis

The diagnosis and treatment of depression in hemodialysis are crucial because untreated depression is associated with poor adherence to management, increased morbidity and mortality rates, and a low quality of life among people undergoing hemodialysis. Generally, the management of depression has been classified into pharmacological and nonpharmacological interventions. Management approaches should be adapted to the patient's unique needs (e.g., treatment history, concurrent illnesses, and preferences of the patients and their family) and consider the resources available in the dialysis facilities [38].

3.2.1 Pharmacological treatment

Antidepressant drugs have been shown to be effective in treating depression in the general population [64]. However, in dialysis, this is still ambiguous. For safety concerns and the possibility of serious adverse events, there are few antidepressant trials conducted among hemodialysis patients to support their efficiency. The pharmacokinetics of antidepressant drugs in hemodialysis are likely to be affected due to several factors. In fact, the metabolism of antidepressant drugs is such that these drugs frequently go through the liver, and the active metabolites are eliminated by the kidneys instead [38]. Impaired kidney functions negatively influence the excretion process, which causes buildup toxic concentrations of the drug in the body. In addition, since antidepressants are typically heavily protein bound, dialysis does not significantly eliminate them from the body [38, 64]. Moreover, there is a high risk of drug-drug interactions in dialysis patients due to the polypharmacy taken for the treatment of kidney failure and associated comorbidities [38].

The selective serotonin reuptake inhibitors (SSRIs) are the most common antidepressant drugs to use [36]. In hemodialysis, the SSRIs are still under debate [36, 65].

Both meta-analyses and a recent systematic review revealed that the evidence related to SSRIs is not sufficient, and the findings are contradictory [66, 67]. Some placebo-controlled trials show low or ungradable benefits [66, 67]. Among the SSRIs, fluoxetine is the most researched, with a daily dose of 20–60 mg considered tolerable [16, 68]. Another review has focused on the use of sertraline in hemodialysis and found that the use of sertraline appears to be safe but needs more investigation [69]. A double-blind randomized clinical trial found that sertraline has improved pruritis intensity in hemodialysis patients [70]. Other examples of drugs in the same class are citalopram, escitalopram, fluvoxamine, and paroxetine. Despite the fact that there is insufficient evidence to support the efficacy of SSRIs in hemodialysis patients, they have fewer anticholinergic and cardiac side effects than other drugs, such as tricyclic antidepressants (TCAs), which adds to their privilege [65]. Further, a recent systematic review found that side effects for SSRIs were minor, such as fatigue and nausea [66]. Another reported side effect of SSRIs is an increased risk of bleeding, which requires cautious use in patients with platelet dysfunction [16]. Importantly, patients should be observed for any suicide attempts, as a risk of suicide during the SSRI treatment may potentially occur during the initial administration [39]. The initial treatment should be started with a low dose, and the clinical effects should be monitored closely for at least 4–6 months [16]. If the result is suboptimal, the dose may be increased or the drug changed [16, 65].

Selective norepinephrine reuptake inhibitors, such as venlafaxine and bupropion hydrochloride, are examples of a different class of antidepressants that are also used with caution [16, 39]. Monoamine oxidase inhibitors are used, but not preferred as they have many side effects, especially hypotension [16]. **Table 1** summarizes the antidepressant drug classes and recommended dosing in patients undergoing hemodialysis [68].

We should notice that depression could happen due to multiple factors, including triggers of other symptoms such as fatigue, sleep disturbance, and sexual dysfunction [71–74]. Given this, clinicians should comprehensively assess the potential correlating factors before prescribing any antidepressant medications. The possible management of depression may be conducted indirectly through the management of the source of the issue.

3.2.2 Nonpharmacological interventions

The optimal care to enhance mental health includes nonpharmacological interventions as a key component to reduce stress, improve cognitive function, and enhance coping. Nonpharmacological interventions have been considered due to safety concerns and a lack of evidence about the efficacy of pharmacological regimens for depression in hemodialysis patients. In contrast, many studies have shown that using these alternative approaches has significant clinical outcomes in the treatment of depression in hemodialysis patients [75–79]. These include cognitive behavioral therapy (CBT), psychoeducation, exercise programmers, relaxation training, acupuncture therapy, self-management, problem-solving, meditation and laughter therapies, and mindfulness-based stress reduction [36, 38, 66, 68, 80].

Cognitive behavioral therapy (CBT) is a common psychotherapy approach to depression treatment. The main principle of CBT focuses on resolving the cognitive factors that lead to psychological distress, such as coping and acceptance. It is based on an organized approach to encourage the restructuring of negative ideas, improve mental status, and enhance behavioral adaptations [68]. A growing body of evidence supports

Medication class	Medication	Recommended dose	Class adverse effects
Monoamine oxidase inhibitor	Isocarboxacid	30–60 mg daily, in single or divided doses	Significant drug-drug interactions, risk of hypertensive crisis with tyramine-rich food, orthostatic hypotension
	Phenelzine	45–90 mg daily, in three divided doses	
	Tranylcypromine	30 mg daily, increase with caution	
	Selegiline	5 mg daily	
Tricyclic antidepressants	Clomipramine	10 mg daily, increase with caution	Prolonged QT syndrome, arrhythmias, orthostatic hypotension, central nervous system and anticholinergic effects
	Desipramine	25 mg daily, increase with caution	
	Lofepramine	140 mg daily, in two divided doses, increase with caution	
	Nortriptyline	30–150 mg daily, in single of divided doses	
	Amitriptyline	75–200 mg daily	
	Amitriptylinoxide	15–150 mg daily	
	Dibenzepine	240 mg daily, increase with caution	
	Dosulepine	75 mg daily, increase with caution	
	Doxepine	10–300 mg daily, maximal single dose 100 mg	
	Imipramine	10 mg daily, increase with caution	
	Protriptyline	15 mg daily, increase with caution	
	Mianserin	30 mg daily, increase with caution	
	Amoxapine	75–400 mg daily, in single or divided doses	
	Maprotiline	50 mg daily, increase with caution	
Selective serotonin reuptake inhibitors	Citalopram	10–40 mg daily	Increased risk of bleeding, nausea, diarrheal, central nervous system effects, sexual dysfunction
	Escitalopram	10 mg, increase with caution	
	Fluvoxamine	50–300 mg daily, maximal single dose 150 mg	
	Fluoxetine	20-60 mg daily	
	Paroxetine	10 mg daily, increase with caution	
	Sertraline	25 mg daily	

Medication class	Medication	Recommended dose	Class adverse effects
Serotonin/ norepinephrine reuptake inhibitors	Venlafaxine	37.5–112.5 mg daily, in three divided doses	Hypertension, sexual dysfunction, neuroleptic malignant syndrome, serotonin syndrome
	Desvenlafaxine	25 mg daily	
	Duloxetine	40 mg daily, increase with caution	
	Milnacipran	25–50 mg daily	
Serotonin modulators	Nefazodone	100 mg daily, increase with caution	Cardiac dysrhythmias, Steven-Johnson syndrome, liver failure, serotonin syndrome, priapism
	Trazodone	150 mg daily, increase with caution	
Noradrenergic and serotonergic agonist	Mirtazapine	15 mg daily, increase with caution	Central nervous systems effects including somnolence, weight gain
Norepinephrine dopamine reuptake inhibitors	Bupropion	150 mg daily	Accumulation of toxic metabolites, cardiac dysrhythmia, wide QRS complex, nausea, insomnia, dizziness
Dopamine receptor agonist	Trimipramine	150 mg daily, increase with caution	Sedation (especially common with trimipramine compared to the other tricyclics), anticholinergic effects
Reversible monoamine oxidase inhibitor	Moclobemide	300–600 mg daily, in three divided doses	Nausea, dry mouth, constipation, insomnia, dizziness, anxiety, restlessness
Selective serotonin re-uptake enhancer	Tianeptine	12.5–25 mg daily	Insomnia, dry mouth, nausea, headache, constipation, drowsiness, weight gain
Melatonergic antidepressant	Agomelatine	5–50 mg daily	Sweating, gastrointestinal side effects, insomnia, anxiety, elevated liver enzymes
Selective norepinephrine reuptake inhibitor	Reboxetine	4–6 mg daily, in 2–3 divided doses	Insomnia, dry mouth, nausea constipation, sweating, tachycardia

Adapted from Ma et al. with permission [68].

Table 1.
Antidepressant medication classes and dosing in dialysis patients.

the clinical effectiveness of CBT for depression management in hemodialysis. Eight randomized placebo-controlled trials examining the efficacy of CBT were examined in a meta-analysis study, and the results showed that CBT was successful in easing depressive symptoms in hemodialysis patients [81]. However, this approach requires face-to-face psychotherapeutic intervention, which may be difficult for this population. Therefore, it has been suggested that internet-delivered self-help CBT (ICBT) would be a promising approach to the management of depression [82]. Other proposed nonpharmacological interventions yet need further investigation to draw conclusions about their efficacy.

4. Anxiety

Anxiety is another frequent and overlooked psychiatric disorder in patients undergoing hemodialysis. Less clinical attention has been given to anxiety in hemodialysis compared with depression [39]. It is defined as anticipation of a potential danger or threat [83]. Anxiety is an emotional condition characterized by excessive nervousness, fear, worry, and tension [84]. It may also cause physiological manifestations such as sweating and an increase in heart rate and blood pressure. According to American Psychiatric Association, there are different types of anxiety disorder, which include generalized anxiety, panic disorder, phobia, agoraphobia, social anxiety disorder, and separation anxiety disorder (**Table 2**), [84]. When anxiety exceeds what would be predicted given a usual response to a certain incident, its severity and duration are considered disorders. Most anxiety disorders have a minimum 6-month duration, and the severity is considered excessive compared with the real level of threat [83]. Studies have found that anxiety is often associated with depression [80, 85]. Thus, other psychiatric disorders (e.g., depression and post-traumatic stress disorder) may display anxiety as a diagnostic sign [83].

Type	Characteristics
Generalized anxiety	• Persistent and excessive worry for at least six months • Beside the psychological symptoms, it involves physical symptoms, such as restlessness, difficulty concentrating, muscle tension, or sleep issues.
Panic disorder	• Involve recurrent, sudden panic attacks • Combine extremely distressing physical and mental symptoms
Phobia	• Excessive and persistent fear of a specific object, situation, or activity
Agoraphobia	• Fear of being in circumstances where getting out would be challenging or embarrassing, or where getting aid might be difficult in the event of panic attacks. This extreme fear appears in two or more of the following situations: • Using public transportation • Being in open spaces • Being in close places • Standing in line or being in a crowd • Bing outside the home alone
Social anxiety disorder	• It is associated with intense worry and discomfort about social activities and situations. The worry or anxiety lasts for at least six months and interferes with daily functioning.
Separation anxiety disorder	• Excessively nervous or afraid of being parted from persons to whom they are attached.

Table 2.
Types of anxiety disorder.

4.1 Screening and diagnostic measures

There are limited studies reporting the prevalence of anxiety and its associated factors among patients undergoing hemodialysis. Anxiety prevalence ranges from 25.9–50% [20, 80, 85–87]. The discrepancy in range is probably due to variations in the applied methodology for screening for anxiety and the diversity of patient populations. Some studies rely on a general measure designed for symptom assessment that includes anxiety as one component, such as the Dialysis Symptom Index and the Chronic Kidney Disease Symptom Burden Index [88, 89]. Others use specific measures for anxiety assessment, such as HADS, the Beck Anxiety Inventory, and the Primary Care Evaluation of Mental Disorders (PRIME-MD). The BAI contains 21 items based on a 4-point Likert scale that examine the severity of anxiety [90]. Each question is scored between 0 (not at all) and 3 (severely it bothered me a lot). A high score suggests an increased level of anxiety symptoms. Low anxiety is indicated by a score between 0 and 21. A score range of 22–35 indicates moderate anxiety, while a score of 36 or above indicates a severe anxiety level [90]. The BAI is a valid and reliable measure. The psychometric analysis showed a high level of internal consistency, and the discrimination validity of the scale was demonstrated when it differentiated between those who were anxious and those who were not anxious but had other psychiatric issues, such as depression [90]. Numerous studies used the BAI to assess anxiety levels among patients undergoing hemodialysis [91–94]. Nadort et al. compared the diagnostic accuracy of BAI and HADS and concluded that both scales were valid for anxiety screening in hemodialysis but that HADS is more useful in routine dialysis care [95]. Regarding the PRIME-MD, it is one of the primary screening tools for mental health. It consists of two parts. The first part is a one-page questionnaire (PQ) that should be filled out by the patient, and the second part is a 12-page clinician evaluation guide that should be completed by clinicians using a structured interview form [96]. The PRIME-MD-PQ is a self-administered tool that contains 26 questions based on yes/no choices regarding the existence of symptoms related to mood, anxiety, somatoform, eating disorders, and alcohol abuse [96]. Some studies use the PRIME-MD to assess anxiety in hemodialysis [97, 98].

A semistructured clinical interview was also used for anxiety diagnosis. The prevalence of moderate-to-high levels of anxiety is reported at 35.9%, with 17.1% reporting a high level of anxiety [80]. A prior study that surveyed 395 hemodialysis patients in Greece using HADS found that 47.8% of patients suffer from anxiety [20]. Similarly, a study conducted in Saudi Arabia using the same instrument found that the prevalence of anxiety was 50% [85].

On a dialysis unit, there are numerous factors that could stimulus anxiety; for instance, cannulation in hemodialysis, dialysis machine alarms, lack of control over treatment, and feeling dependent [99, 100]. Anxiety has a significant negative effect on the quality of life of hemodialysis patients [85, 93, 101]. It is correlated with negative clinical results, for example, increased hospitalization frequency and length of stay and high mortality rates [93]. Sometimes, it can influence the ability to focus and the way to process information. This may cause some disruptive behaviors that contradict healthcare professionals [83].

4.2 Management of anxiety in hemodialysis

Treatment options for anxiety are similar to those for depression and include both nonpharmacological and pharmacological treatments. The nonpharmacological interventions include psychotherapy and cognitive behavioral therapy. Furthermore, using relaxation techniques is a useful method to reduce anxiety in hemodialysis patients [80]. Prior research found the effectiveness of Benson relaxation training in reducing the level of anxiety among eighty patients on hemodialysis [102]. A recent systematic review that examined the benefit of Benson relaxation training in managing anxiety on hemodialysis found that Benson relaxation was an effective method of management [103]. A randomized controlled trial that was implemented to examine the effectiveness of acupressure therapy in patients receiving hemodialysis also found a significant reduction in anxiety levels [104]. Apart from these methods, the social support derived from family, clinicians, and the community can improve psychological status and alleviate anxiety [80].

If those methods were unsuccessful, different types of medications could be used. Short-acting benzodiazepines (e.g., lorazepam or alprazolam) are recommended for limited periods at low doses. From this class, lbrium (chlordiazepoxide) and valium (diazepam) should be avoided in patients undergoing hemodialysis [16]. In a severely anxious patient, antipsychotic medications (e.g., haloperidol) may be clinically feasible [16]. However, there is still window for future studies to explore the best management options for anxiety in hemodialysis.

5. Delirium

Delirium is a neurocognitive disorder characterized by an acute episode of confusion of memory, awareness, and thinking [65]. It is often a reversible state among patients undergoing maintenance hemodialysis. It could occur owing to a medical condition, uremia, intoxication, or drug adverse effect. Moreover, studies suggest that this disorder is more prevalent among elderly patients [65, 105]. A recent study found that delirium is independently associated with early mortality in the elderly after starting hemodialysis [106]. The acute delirium could lead to self-harm and death [107].

A rare kind of delirium in hemodialysis is dialysis disequilibrium syndrome, which is a serious form of complication. Headache, visual disturbance, nausea, and agitation are common symptoms of the syndrome, and in more serious cases, delirium, lethargy, seizures, or even coma may also occur [65]. It was noted during or following the initial round of dialysis. Additionally, long-term hemodialysis has increased reports of dialysis disequilibrium syndrome [65].

5.1 Screening and diagnostic measures

Nurses and physicians should be on the lookout for any signs of delirium and screen their patients for any changes in cognition or behavior. Any concerns or suspicions of delirium should be investigated further using a validated tool. The Confusion Assessment Method (CAM) is one of the most valuable tools for detecting delirium. It is designed to help medical professionals without backgrounds in psychiatry or mental health and recognize patients with delirium quickly in high-risk situations [108]. The assessment includes questions that aim to assess delirium through four criteria: (1) acute onset and fluctuating course; (2) intention; (3) disorganized thinking; and (4) altered level of consciousness. The CAM algorithm for the diagnosis of delirium requires having criteria 1 and 2 and either 3 or 4 [108]. Other available tools to assess delirium include the Mini-Mental State Examination. As nurses provide frequent direct care for patients on hemodialysis, assessment of delirium using a validated tool should be integrated into renal nursing care for early detection of delirium.

5.2 Management of delirium in hemodialysis

Starting hemodialysis slowly and gently, using a high dialysate sodium concentration and adding osmotic agents (sodium, mannitol, and glucose) to the blood stream are all ways to avoid delirium in hemodialysis [109]. Other preventive measures include active communication with the patient, avoiding medication interactions, maintaining hydration, and managing the pain [65].

Management of underlying factors is a key for management of delirium [65]. Supportive management provided as appropriate to prevent aspiration and pressure sores. When delirium endangers patient safety or interferes with crucial treatments, pharmacologic treatment is necessary [65]. Antipsychotic medications, such as haloperidol, are drug of choice in the beginning. Benzodiazepines and some antidepressants have also been used for treatment of delirium. The management of underlying factors is critical in the treatment of delirium [65]. Supportive management is provided as appropriate to prevent aspiration and pressure sores. When delirium endangers patients' safety or interferes with crucial treatments, pharmacologic treatment is necessary [65]. In the beginning, haloperidol from antipsychotic medication is considered a drug of choice. Treatment for delirium has also included the use of benzodiazepines and various antidepressants drugs. Dialysis should be stopped in cases of seizure until vital signs stabilize [109].

6. Withdrawal from dialysis

It is known that the leading cause of death in dialysis is associated with cardiovascular disease and infection. Psychosocial factors are also concerning factors that contribute to death in dialysis patients. Withdrawal from dialysis results in death due to the clinical manifestations of uremia caused by treatment discontinuation. In dialysis patients, withdrawal is categorized as the third-most frequent reason for mortality [110]. In Western countries, the incidence of withdrawal from dialysis prior to death ranges from 20–30% [8, 111–113]. In North America, the incidence of withdrawal from dialysis accounts for 30% of deaths before death [114]. The decision to discontinue dialysis is associated with several factors, such as older age, female gender, white race, and clinical complications [115–118]. A retrospective cohort study of 133,162 hemodialysis incidents found that 10% of patients who withdrew from dialysis were 80 years of age or older [117]. The psychosocial risk factors that could be associated with increased odds of withdrawal from dialysis are depression, low socioeconomic status, and dementia [39, 110, 117, 119]. Furthermore, the most common reasons for considering dialysis withdrawal in many cases are a lack of enjoyment in life, a sense of being a burden on others, a shift in roles, a loss of control, and lack of social support [114]. Also, studies suggest that high symptom burden, such as pain, is associated with withdrawal from dialysis [114, 120]. There are several obstacles in the process of withdrawal from dialysis that relate to patient and family preferences, cultural and religious views, ethical and legal issues, and priorities in policymaking [114].

6.1 Prevention of withdrawal from dialysis

Indeed, it is important to early recognize those who are at high risk for withdrawal from dialysis to provide them with other solutions, eliminate the potential barriers, and facilitate taking an informed decision. Nurses and physicians are well positioned to provide early intervention for underlying factors, to educate patients about their care, and to provide a comprehensive approach to care. Regardless of the patient's decision, it is unethical to leave patients after their withdrawal from dialysis to suffer from pain and other complications. Since the beginning of their treatment, patients on dialysis and their families should be informed about the possibility of withdrawal from dialysis and the consequences of this option [121]. Therefore, clinicians can offer a good palliative and end-of-life care by alleviating the symptoms and pain management.

7. Conclusion

There are various psychosocial issues that are associated with hemodialysis therapy. There are various psychosocial issues that are associated with hemodialysis therapy. These issues may arise at any stage of the trajectory of hemodialysis. Some issues occur during the initial transition period of hemodialysis; others occur after a long time of receiving hemodialysis or after changing the modality of treatment. Examples of these issues are depression, anxiety, delirium, and withdrawal from dialysis. Due to the complexity of hemodialysis and its accompanying symptoms, identifying these issues remains difficult. This chapter has summarized the most common psychosocial issues among patients undergoing hemodialysis. The early recognition of the high-risk group developing some of these issues in hemodialysis is important for early management, which is cost-effective. Using short screening methods is applicable in clinical practice. Furthermore, for safety concerns, it is recommended to initiate management with nonpharmacological interventions. If the issues are still persistent or there is no improvement, pharmacology-based intervention might be the solution, but with caution.

Conflict of interest

The authors declare no conflict of interest.

Author details

Hayfa Almutary
King Abdulaziz University, Jeddah, Saudi Arabia

*Address all correspondence to: aalalmetere2@kau.edu.sa

References

[1] White Y, Grenyer BF. The biopsychosocial impact of end-stage renal disease: The experience of dialysis patients and their partners. Journal of Advanced Nursing. 1999;**30**(6):1312-1320. DOI: 10.1046/j.1365-2648.1999.01236.x

[2] Montalescot L, Rascle N, Combe C, Untas A. Patients' experience one year after dialysis initiation: A lexicometric analysis. Health Psychology and Behavioral Medicine. 2021;**9**(1):380-397. DOI: https://www.tandfonline.com/loi/rhpb20

[3] Schell JO, Patel UD, Steinhauser KE, Ammarell N, Tulsky JA. Discussions of the kidney disease trajectory by elderly patients and nephrologists: A qualitative study. American Journal of Kidney Diseases. 2012;**59**(4):495-503. DOI: 10.1053/j.ajkd.2011.11.023

[4] Harwood L, Locking-Cusolito H, Spittal J, Wilson B, White S. Preparing for hemodialysis: Patient stressors and responses. Nephrology Nursing Journal. 2005;**32**(3):295-302

[5] Reid C, Seymour J, Jones C. A thematic synthesis of the experiences of adults living with hemodialysis. Clinical Journal of the American Society of Nephrology. 2016;**11**(7):1206-1218. DOI: 10.2215/CJN.10561015

[6] Offer D, Offer MK, Szafir SO. Dialysis Without Fear: A Guide to Living Well on Dialysis for Patients and Their Families. New York: Oxford University Press; 2007

[7] Nowak Z, Wańkowicz Z, Laudanski K. Denial defense mechanism in dialyzed patients. Medical Science Monitor: International Medical Journal of Experimental and Clinical Research. 2015;**21**:1798. DOI: 10.12659/MSM.893331

[8] Ellwood AD, Jassal SV, Suri RS, Clark WF, Na Y, Moist LM. Early dialysis initiation and rates and timing of withdrawal from dialysis in Canada. Clinical Journal of the American Society of Nephrology. 2013;**8**(2):265-270. DOI: 10.2215/CJN.01000112

[9] Kim MH, Kim YC, Lee JP, Kim H, Kim DK, Ryu DR, et al. Three-year income trends in Korean adults commencing haemodialysis: A prospective cohort. Nephrology. 2018;**23**(7):625-632. DOI: 10.1111/nep.13065

[10] Manen van JG, Korevaar JC, Dekker FW, Reuselaars MC, Boeschoten EW, Krediet RT. Changes in employment status in end-stage renal disease patients during their first year of dialysis. Peritoneal Dialysis International. 2001;**21**(6):595-601. DOI: 10.1177/089686080102100610

[11] Allen K, Damery SL, Sein K, Johnson DW, Davies SJ, Lambie M, et al. How do patients and their family members experience the transition from peritoneal dialysis to incentre haemodialysis? A multisite qualitative study in England and Australia. Peritoneal Dialysis International. 2022;**42**(3):297-304. DOI: 10.1177/0896860820975596

[12] American Psychiatric Association. What is Depression [Internet]. 2022. Available from: https://www.psychiatry.org/patients-families/depression/what-is-depression

[13] Davison GC, Neale JM. Abnormal Psychology. 8th ed. New York: John Wiley; 2004

[14] National Institute of Mental Health. Depression [Internet]. 2022. Available

from: https://www.nimh.nih.gov/health/topics/depression. [Accessed: November 12, 2022]

[15] American Psychiatric Association. Diagnostic and Statistical Manual of Mental Disorders. 5th ed. Arlington, VA: American Psychiatric Publishing; 2013

[16] Cohen SD, Cukor D, Kimmel PL. Psychosocial issues. In: Daugirdas JT, Blake PG, Ing TS, editors. Handbook of Dialysis. 5th ed. Philadelphia: Wolters Kluwer; 2015. pp. 528-534

[17] Kim B, Kim J. Influence of uncertainty, depression, and social support on self-care compliance in hemodialysis patients. Therapeutics and Clinical Risk Management. 2019;**15**:1243. DOI: 10.2147/TCRM.S218934

[18] Ok E, Kutlu FY. Hopelessness, anxiety, depression and treatment adherence in chronic hemodialysis patients. International Journal of Caring Sciences. 2019;**12**(1):423-429

[19] Schouten RW, Harmse VJ, Dekker FW, van Ballegooijen W, Siegert CE, Honig A. Dimensions of depressive symptoms and their association with mortality, hospitalization, and quality of life in dialysis patients: A cohort study. Psychosomatic Medicine. 2019;**81**(7):649. DOI: 10.1097/PSY.0000000000000723

[20] Vasilopoulou C, Bourtsi E, Giaple S, Koutelekos I, Theofilou P, Polikandrioti M. The impact of anxiety and depression on the quality of life of hemodialysis patients. Global Journal of Health Science. 2016;**8**(1):45. DOI: 10.5539/gjhs.v8n1p45

[21] Wang HH, Ho MC, Hung KY, Cheng HT. A single question regarding mobility in the World Health Organization quality of life questionnaire predicts 3-year mortality in patients receiving chronic hemodialysis. Scientific Reports. 2017;**7**(1):10. DOI: 10.1038/s41598-017-12276-9

[22] Clarke DM, Currie KC. Depression, anxiety and their relationship with chronic diseases: A review of the epidemiology, risk and treatment evidence. The Medical Journal of Australia. 2009;**190**:S54-S60

[23] Lin J, Ye H, Yi C, Li J, Yu X, Zhu L, et al. The negative impact of depressive symptoms on patient and technique survival in peritoneal dialysis: A prospective cohort study. International Urology and Nephrology. 2020;**52**(12):2393-2401. DOI: 10.1007/s11255-020-02593-w

[24] Tsai YC, Chiu YW, Hung CC, Hwang SJ, Tsai JC, Wang SL, et al. Association of symptoms of depression with progression of CKD. American Journal of Kidney Diseases. 2012;**60**(1):54-61. DOI: 10.1053/j.ajkd.2012.02.325

[25] Cheng HT, Ho MC, Hung KY. Affective and cognitive rather than somatic symptoms of depression predict 3-year mortality in patients on chronic hemodialysis. Scientific Reports. 2018;**8**(1):1-2. DOI: 10.1038/s41598-018-24267-5

[26] World Health Organization. Depression. [Internet]. 2022. Available from: https://www.who.int/news-room/fact-sheets/detail/depression#:~:text=Globally%2C%20it%20is%20estimated%20that,overall%20global%20burden%20of%20disease. [Accessed: November 12, 2022]

[27] Zalai D, Szeifert L, Novak M. Psychological distress and depression in patients with chronic kidney disease. In: Seminars in Dialysis 2012. Oxford, UK: Blackwell Publishing Ltd

[28] Palmer S, Vecchio M, Craig JC, Tonelli M, Johnson DW, Nicolucci A, et al. Prevalence of depression in chronic kidney disease: Systematic review and meta-analysis of observational studies. Kidney International. 2013;**84**(1):179-191. DOI: 10.1038/ki.2013.77

[29] Shirazian S, Grant CD, Aina O, Mattana J, Khorassani F, Ricardo AC. Depression in chronic kidney disease and end-stage renal disease: Similarities and differences in diagnosis, epidemiology, and management. Kidney International Reports. 2017;**2**(1):94-107. DOI: 10.1016/j.ekir.2016.09.005

[30] Haverkamp GL, Loosman WL, Schouten RW, Franssen CF, Kema IP, van Diepen M, et al. Longitudinal associations between inflammation and depressive symptoms in chronic dialysis patients. Psychosomatic Medicine. 2019;**81**(1):74-80. DOI: 10.1097/PSY.0000000000000649

[31] Lacson E Jr, Li NC, Guerra-Dean S, Lazarus M, Hakim R, Finkelstein FO. Depressive symptoms associate with high mortality risk and dialysis withdrawal in incident hemodialysis patients. Nephrology, Dialysis, Transplantation. 2012;**27**(7):2921-2928. DOI: 10.1093/ndt/gfr778

[32] Bautovich A, Katz I, Loo CK, Harvey SB. Beck depression inventory as a screening tool for depression in chronic haemodialysis patients. Australasian Psychiatry. 2018;**26**(3):281-284. DOI: 10.1177/1039856218758582

[33] Saglimbene V, Palmer S, Scardapane M, Craig JC, Ruospo M, Natale P, et al. Depression and all-cause and cardiovascular mortality in patients on haemodialysis: A multinational cohort study. Nephrology, Dialysis, Transplantation. 2017;**32**(2):377-384. DOI: 10.1093/ndt/gfw016

[34] Almutary H. Depression, sleep disturbance, and quality of life in patients undergoing dialysis therapy. Applied Nursing Research. 2022;**67**:151610. DOI: 10.1016/j.apnr.2022.151610

[35] Sallam L, Alsharif F, Abaalalaa S, Alakeely R, Abdullah Z, Alkhamis Z, et al. Prevalence of depression in patients with end-stage renal disease undergoing hemodialysis in Saudi Arabia: A cross-sectional study. Belitung Nursing Journal. 2022;**8**(4):296-303. DOI: 10.33546/bnj.2080

[36] Tian N, Chen N, Li PK. Depression in dialysis. Current Opinion in Nephrology and Hypertension. 2021;**30**(6):600-612. DOI: 10.1097/MNH.0000000000000741

[37] Kondo K, Antick JR, Ayers CK, Kansagara D, Chopra P. Depression screening tools for patients with kidney failure: A systematic review. Clinical Journal of the American Society of Nephrology. 2020;**15**(12):1785-1795. DOI: 10.2215/CJN.05540420

[38] Hedayati SS, Yalamanchili V, Finkelstein FO. A practical approach to the treatment of depression in patients with chronic kidney disease and end-stage renal disease. Kidney International. 2012;**81**(3):247-255. DOI: 10.1038/ki.2011.358

[39] Cukor D, Cohen SD, Peterson RA, Kimmel PL. Psychosocial aspects of chronic disease: ESRD as a paradigmatic illness. Journal of the American Society of Nephrology. 2007;**18**(12):3042-3055. DOI: 10.1681/ASN.2007030345

[40] Weisbord SD, Fried LF, Unruh ML, Kimmel PL, Switzer GE, Fine MJ, et al. Associations of race with depression and symptoms in patients on maintenance haemodialysis. Nephrology, Dialysis, Transplantation. 2007;**22**(1):203-208. DOI: 10.1093/ndt/gfl521

[41] Beck AT, Steer RA, Ball R, Ranieri WF. Comparison of Beck depression inventories-IA and-II in psychiatric outpatients. Journal of Personality Assessment. 1996;**67**(3):588-597. DOI: 10.1207/s15327752jpa6703_13

[42] Jackson-Koku G. Beck depression inventory. Occupational Medicine. 2016;**66**(2):174-175. DOI: 10.1093/occmed/kqv087

[43] Hedayati SS, Minhajuddin AT, Toto RD, Morris DW, Rush AJ. Validation of depression screening scales in patients with CKD. American Journal of Kidney Diseases. 2009;**54**(3):433-439. DOI: 10.1053/j.ajkd.2009.03.016

[44] Gregg LP, Hedayati SS. Screening for depression in people with kidney failure. Clinical Journal of the American Society of Nephrology. 2020;**15**(12):1702-1704. DOI: 10.2215/CJN.16381020

[45] Nah R, Robertson N, Niyi-Odumosu FA, Clarke AL, Bishop NC, Smith AC. Relationships between illness representations, physical activity and depression in chronic kidney disease. Journal of Renal Care. 2019;**45**(2):74-82. DOI: 10.1111/jorc.12274

[46] Naja S, Al-Kubaisi N, Chehab M, Al-Dahshan A, Abuhashem N, Bougmiza I. Psychometric properties of the Arabic version of EPDS and BDI-II as a screening tool for antenatal depression: Evidence from Qatar. BMJ Open. 2019;**9**(9):e030365. DOI: 10.1136/bmjopen-2019-030365

[47] Rajan EJ, Subramanian S. The effect of depression and anxiety on the performance status of end-stage renal disease patients undergoing hemodialysis. Saudi Journal of Kidney Diseases and Transplantation. 2016;**27**(2):331. DOI: 10.4103/1319-2442.178555

[48] Tu CY, Chou YH, Lin YH, Huang WL. Sleep and emotional disturbance in patients with non-dialysis chronic kidney disease. Journal of the Formosan Medical Association. 2019;**118**(6):986-994. DOI: 10.1016/j.jfma.2018.10.016

[49] Tuot DS, Lin F, Norris K, Gassman J, Smogorzewski M, Ku E. Depressive symptoms associate with race and all-cause mortality in patients with CKD. Kidney international reports. 2019;**4**(2):222-230. DOI: 10.1016/j.ekir.2018.10.001

[50] Neitzer A, Sun S, Doss S, Moran J, Schiller B. Beck Depression Inventory-Fast Screen (BDI-FS): An efficient tool for depression screening in patients with end-stage renal disease. Hemodialysis International. 2012;**16**(2):207-213. DOI: 10.1111/j.1542-4758.2012.00663.x

[51] Sacks CR, Peterson RA, Kimmel PL. Perception of illness and depression in chronic renal disease. American Journal of Kidney Diseases. 1990;**15**(1):31-39. DOI: 10.1016/S0272-6386(12)80589-0

[52] Kimmel PL, Peterson RA, Weihs KL, Simmens SJ, Alleyne S, Cruz I, et al. Multiple measurements of depression predict mortality in a longitudinal study of chronic hemodialysis outpatients. Kidney International. 2000;**57**(5):2093-2098. DOI: 10.1046/j.1523-1755.2000.00059.x

[53] Peterson RA, Kimmel PL, Sacks CR, Mesquita ML, Simmens SJ, Reiss D. Depression, perception of illness and mortality in patients with end-stage renal disease. The International Journal of Psychiatry in Medicine. 1991;**21**(4):343-354. DOI: 10.2190/D7VA-FWEU-JN5Y-TD3E

[54] Kroenke K, Spitzer RL, Williams JB. The PHQ-9: Validity of a brief depression severity measure. Journal of General Internal

Medicine. 2001;**16**(9):606-613. DOI: 10.1046/j.1525-1497.2001.016009606.x

[55] Watnick S, Wang PL, Demadura T, Ganzini L. Validation of 2 depression screening tools in dialysis patients. American Journal of Kidney Diseases. 2005;**46**(5):919-924. DOI: 10.1053/j.ajkd.2005.08.006

[56] Zigmond AS, Snaith RP. The hospital anxiety and depression scale. Acta Psychiatrica Scandinavica. 1983;**67**(6):361-370. DOI: 10.1111/j.1600-0447.1983.tb09716.x

[57] Alshogran OY, Altawalbeh SM, Khalil AA. Comparison of two self-report scales to assess anxiety and depressive symptoms in hemodialysis patients. Archives of Psychiatric Nursing. 2022;**41**:208-213. DOI: 10.1016/j.apnu.2022.08.004

[58] Ottaviani AC, Betoni LC, Pavarini SC, Gramani Say K, Zazzetta MS, Orlandi FD. Association between anxiety and depression and quality of life of chronic renal patients on hemodialysis. Texto & Contexto-Enfermagem. 2016;**18**:25. DOI: 10.1590/0104-07072016000650015

[59] Semaan V, Noureddine S, Farhood L. Prevalence of depression and anxiety in end-stage renal disease: A survey of patients undergoing hemodialysis. Applied Nursing Research. 2018;**43**:80-85. DOI: 10.1016/j.apnr.2018.07.009

[60] Terkawi AS, Tsang S, AlKahtani GJ, Al-Mousa SH, Al Musaed S, AlZoraigi US, et al. Development and validation of Arabic version of the hospital anxiety and depression scale. Saudi Journal of Anaesthesia. 2017;**11**(5):11

[61] Turkistani I, Nuqali A, Badawi M, Taibah O, Alserihy O, Morad M, et al. The prevalence of anxiety and depression among end-stage renal disease patients on hemodialysis in Saudi Arabia. Renal Failure. 2014;**36**(10):1510-1515. DOI: 10.3109/0886022X.2014.949761

[62] Radloff LS. The CES-D scale: A self-report depression scale for research in the general population. Applied Psychological Measurement. 1977;**1**(3):385-401. DOI: 10.1177/014662167700100306

[63] Agganis BT, Weiner DE, Giang LM, Scott T, Tighiouart H, Griffith JL, et al. Depression and cognitive function in maintenance hemodialysis patients. American Journal of Kidney Diseases. 2010;**56**(4):704-712. DOI: 10.1053/j.ajkd.2010.04.018

[64] Nagler EV, Webster AC, Vanholder R, Zoccali C. Antidepressants for depression in stage 3-5 chronic kidney disease: A systematic review of pharmacokinetics, efficacy and safety with recommendations by European renal best practice (ERBP). Nephrology, Dialysis, Transplantation. 2012;**27**(10):3736-3745. DOI: 10.1093/ndt/gfs295

[65] Tamura MK. Recognizing delirium, dementia, and depression. In: Coffman TM, editor. Geriatric Nephrology Curriculum. USA: American Society of Nephrology; 2009. pp. 1-6

[66] Chopra P, Ayers CK, Antick JR, Kansagara D, Kondo K. The effectiveness of depression treatment for adults with ESKD: A systematic review. Kidney. 2021;**2**(3):558

[67] Palmer SC, Natale P, Ruospo M, Saglimbene VM, Rabindranath KS, Craig JC, et al. Antidepressants for treating depression in adults with end-stage kidney disease treated with dialysis. Cochrane Database of Systematic Reviews. 2016;**5**:1-40. DOI: 10.1002/14651858.CD004541.pub3

[68] Ma TK, Li PK. Depression in dialysis patients. Nephrology. 2016;**21**(8):639-646. DOI: 10.1111/nep.12742

[69] Kubanek A, Paul P, Przybylak M, Kanclerz K, Rojek JJ, Renke M, et al. Use of sertraline in Hemodialysis patients. Medicina. 2021;**57**(9):949. DOI: 10.3390/medicina57090949

[70] Pakfetrat M, Malekmakan L, Hashemi N, Tadayon T. Sertraline can reduce uremic pruritus in hemodialysis patient: A double blind randomized clinical trial from southern Iran. Hemodialysis International. 2018;**22**(1):103-109. DOI: 10.1111/hdi.12540

[71] Bai YL, Chang YY, Chiou CP, Lee BO. Mediating effects of fatigue on the relationships among sociodemographic characteristics, depression, and quality of life in patients receiving hemodialysis. Nursing & Health Sciences. 2019;**21**(2):231-238. DOI: 10.1111/nhs.12587

[72] Bautovich A, Katz I, Smith M, Loo CK, Harvey SB. Depression and chronic kidney disease: A review for clinicians. The Australian and New Zealand Journal of Psychiatry. 2014;**48**(6):530-541. DOI: 10.1177/0004867414528589

[73] Brys AD, Di Stasio E, Lenaert B, Sanguinetti M, Picca A, Calvani R, et al. Serum interleukin-6 and endotoxin levels and their relationship with fatigue and depressive symptoms in patients on chronic haemodialysis. Cytokine. 2020;**125**:154823

[74] Edwards C, Almeida OP, Ford AH. Obstructive sleep apnea and depression: A systematic review and meta-analysis. Maturitas. 2020;**142**:45-54. DOI: 10.1016/j.maturitas.2020.06.002

[75] Chan R, Dear BF, Titov N, Chow J, Suranyi M. Examining internet-delivered cognitive behaviour therapy for patients with chronic kidney disease on haemodialysis: A feasibility open trial. Journal of Psychosomatic Research. 2016;**89**:78-84. DOI: 10.1016/j.jpsychores.2016.08.012

[76] Cukor D, Ver Halen N, Asher DR, Coplan JD, Weedon J, Wyka KE, et al. Psychosocial intervention improves depression, quality of life, and fluid adherence in hemodialysis. Journal of the American Society of Nephrology. 2014;**25**(1):196-206. DOI: 10.1681/ASN.2012111134

[77] Kalani L, Aghababaeian H, Majidipour N, Alasvand M, Bahrami H, Sabouhi F, et al. The effects of acupressure on severity of depression in hemodialysis patients: A randomized controlled trial. Journal of Advanced Pharmacy Education & Research. 2019;**2019**:9

[78] Rhee SY, Song JK, Hong SC, Choi JW, Jeon HJ, Shin DH, et al. Intradialytic exercise improves physical function and reduces intradialytic hypotension and depression in hemodialysis patients. The Korean Journal of Internal Medicine. 2019;**34**(3):588. DOI: 10.3904/kjim.2017.020

[79] Valsaraj BP, Bhat SM, Latha KS. Cognitive behaviour therapy for anxiety and depression among people undergoing haemodialysis: A randomized control trial. Journal of Clinical and Diagnostic Research: JCDR. 2016;**10**(8):VC06. DOI: 10.7860/JCDR/2016/18959.8383

[80] Gerogianni G, Babatsikou F, Polikandrioti M, Grapsa EJ. Management of anxiety and depression in haemodialysis patients: The role of non-pharmacological methods. International Urology and Nephrology. 2019;**51**(1):113-118. DOI: 10.1007/s11255-018-2022-7

[81] Ng CZ, Tang SC, Chan M, Tran BX, Ho CS, Tam WW, et al. A systematic review and meta-analysis of randomized controlled trials of cognitive behavioral therapy for hemodialysis patients with depression. Journal of Psychosomatic Research. 2019;**126**:109834. DOI: 10.1016/j.jpsychores.2019.109834

[82] Tommel J, Evers AW, van Hamersvelt HW, van Dijk S, Chavannes NH, Wirken L, et al. E-HEalth treatment in Long-term Dialysis (E-HELD): Study protocol for a multicenter randomized controlled trial evaluating personalized internet-based cognitive-behavioral therapy in dialysis patients. Trials. 2022;**23**(1):1-20. DOI: 10.1186/s13063-022-06392-9

[83] Cohen SD, Cukor D, Kimmel PL. Anxiety in patients treated with hemodialysis. Clinical Journal of the American Society of Nephrology. 2016;**11**(12):2250-2255. DOI: 10.2215/CJN.02590316

[84] American Psychiatric Association. Anxiety Disorders [Internet]. 2022. Available from: https://www.psychiatry.org/patients-families/anxiety-disorders/what-are-anxiety-disorders. [Accessed: November 10, 2022]

[85] Al-Nashri F, Almutary H. Impact of anxiety and depression on the quality of life of haemodialysis patients. Journal of Clinical Nursing 2022;31(1-2):220-230. DOI: 10.1111/jocn.15900

[86] Meng Y, Wu HT, Niu JL, Zhang Y, Qin H, Huang LL, et al. Prevalence of depression and anxiety and their predictors among patients undergoing maintenance hemodialysis in Northern China: A cross-sectional study. Renal Failure. 2022;**44**(1):933-944. DOI: 10.1080/0886022X.2022.2077761

[87] Almutary H, Bonner A, Douglas C. Which patients with chronic kidney disease have the greatest symptom burden? A comparative study of advanced CKD stage and dialysis modality. Journal of Renal Care. 2016;**42**(2):73-82. DOI: 10.1111/jorc.12152

[88] Almutary H, Bonner A, Douglas C. Arabic translation, adaptation and modification of the Dialysis symptom index for chronic kidney disease stages four and five. BMC Nephrology. 2015;**16**(1):1-8. DOI: 10.1186/s12882-015-0036-2

[89] Weisbord SD, Fried LF, Arnold RM, Rotondi AJ, Fine MJ, Levenson DJ, et al. Development of a symptom assessment instrument for chronic hemodialysis patients: The Dialysis symptom index. Journal of Pain and Symptom Management. 2004;**27**(3):226-240. DOI: 10.1016/j.jpainsymman.2003.07.004

[90] Beck AT, Epstein N, Brown G, Steer RA. An inventory for measuring clinical anxiety: Psychometric properties. Journal of Consulting and Clinical Psychology. 1988;**56**(6):893. DOI: 10.1037/0022-006X.56.6.893

[91] Işık Ulusoy S, Kal Ö. Relationship among coping strategies, quality of life, and anxiety and depressive disorders in hemodialysis patients. Therapeutic Apheresis and Dialysis. 2020;**24**(2):189-196. DOI: 10.1111/1744-9987.12914

[92] Ozkan Kurtgoz P, Sackan F, Kızılarslanoglu MC, Bilgin O, Guney I. Effect of anxiety on COVID-19 infection in hemodialysis patients. Therapeutic Apheresis and Dialysis. 2022;**26**(4):775-780. DOI: 10.1111/1744-9987.13759

[93] Schouten RW, Haverkamp GL, Loosman WL, Shaw PK, van Ittersum FJ, Smets YF, et al. Anxiety symptoms, mortality, and hospitalization in patients receiving maintenance dialysis: A cohort study. American Journal of Kidney

Diseases. 2019;**74**(2):158-166. DOI: 10.1053/j.ajkd.2019.02.017

[94] Wu YH, Hsu YJ, Tzeng WC. Correlation between physical activity and psychological distress in patients receiving Hemodialysis with comorbidities: A cross-sectional study. International Journal of Environmental Research and Public Health. 2022;**19**(7):3972. DOI: 10.3390/ijerph19073972

[95] Nadort E, van Geenen NJ, Schouten RW, Boeschoten RE, Chandie Shaw P, Vleming LJ, et al. Validation of two screening tools for anxiety in Hemodialysis patients. Journal of Personalized Medicine. 2022;**12**(7):1077. DOI: 10.3390/jpm12071077

[96] Spitzer RL, Williams JB, Kroenke K, Linzer M, deGruy FV, Hahn SR, et al. Utility of a new procedure for diagnosing mental disorders in primary care: The PRIME-MD 1000 study. Journal of the American Medical Association. 1994;**272**(22):1749-1756. DOI: 10.1001/jama.1994.03520220043029

[97] Preljevic VT, Østhus TB, Sandvik L, Bringager CB, Opjordsmoen S, Nordhus IH, et al. Psychiatric disorders, body mass index and C-reactive protein in dialysis patients. General Hospital Psychiatry. 2011;**33**(5):454-461. DOI: 10.1016/j.genhosppsych.2011.06.010

[98] Taskapan H, Ates F, Kaya B, Emul M, Kaya M, Taskapan C, et al. Psychiatric disorders and large interdialytic weight gain in patients on chronic haemodialysis. Nephrology. 2005;**10**(1):15-20. DOI: 10.1111/j.1440-1797.2005.00321.x

[99] Kopple JD, Shapiro BB, Feroze U, Kim JC, Zhang M, Li Y, et al. Hemodialysis treatment engenders anxiety and emotional distress. Clinical Nephrology. 2017;**88**(4):205. DOI: 10.5414/CN109112

[100] Nataatmadja M, Evangelidis N, Manera KE, Cho Y, Johnson DW, Craig JC, et al. Perspectives on mental health among patients receiving dialysis. Nephrology, Dialysis, Transplantation. 2021;**36**(7):1317-1325. DOI: 10.1093/ndt/gfaa346

[101] Olagunju AT, Campbell EA, Adeyemi JD. Interplay of anxiety and depression with quality of life in endstage renal disease. Psychosomatics. 2015;**56**(1):67-77. DOI: 10.1016/j.psym.2014.03.006

[102] Mahdavi A, Gorji MA, Gorji AM, Yazdani J, Ardebil MD. Implementing benson's relaxation training in hemodialysis patients: Changes in perceived stress, anxiety, and depression. North American Journal of Medical Sciences. 2013;**5**(9):536. Available from: https://www.najms.org/text.asp?2013/5/9/536/118917

[103] Abu Maloh HI, Soh KL, AbuRuz ME, Chong SC, Ismail SI, Soh KG, et al. Efficacy of Benson's relaxation technique on anxiety and depression among patients undergoing Hemodialysis: A systematic review. Clinical Nursing Research. 2022;**31**(1):122-135. DOI: 10.1177/10547738211024797

[104] Hmwe NT, Subramanian P, Tan LP, Chong WK. The effects of acupressure on depression, anxiety and stress in patients with hemodialysis: A randomized controlled trial. International Journal of Nursing Studies. 2015;**52**(2):509-518. DOI: 10.1016/j.ijnurstu.2014.11.002

[105] Inouye SK. Delirium in older persons. The New England Journal of Medicine. 2006;**354**(11):1157-1165. DOI: 10.1056/NEJMra052321

[106] Arai Y, Shioji S, Tanaka H, Kondo I, Sakamoto E, Suzuki M, et al. Delirium is independently associated with early mortality in elderly patients starting

hemodialysis. Clinical and Experimental Nephrology. 2020;**24**(11):1077-1083. DOI: 10.1007/s10157-020-01941-5

[107] Brown PA, Magner PO, Hiremath S, Clark EG. Death due to delirium: A case of a self-cut hemodialysis dialysis catheter-a case report. BMC Nephrology. 2019;**20**(1):1-4. DOI: 10.1186/s12882-019-1571-z

[108] Inouye SK, van Dyck CH, Alessi CA, Balkin S, Siegal AP, Horwitz RI. Clarifying confusion: The confusion assessment method: A new method for detection of delirium. Annals of Internal Medicine. 1990;**113**(12):941-948. DOI: 10.7326/0003-4819-113-12-941

[109] Advanced Renal Education Program. Dialysis Disequilibrium Syndrome (DDS). [Internet]. 2020. Available from: https://advancedrenaleducation.com/wparep/article/disequilibriumsyndrome/#:~:text=Disequilibrium%20syndrome%20(DDS)%20is%20a,rarely%2C%20it%20can%20be%20fatal [Accessed: November 24, 2022]

[110] Gelfand SL, Scherer JS, Koncicki HM. Kidney supportive care: Core curriculum 2020. American Journal of Kidney Diseases. 2020;**75**(5):793-806. DOI: 10.1053/j.ajkd.2019.10.016

[111] Findlay MD, Donaldson K, Doyle A, Fox JG, Khan I, McDonald J, et al. Factors influencing withdrawal from dialysis: A national registry study. Nephrology, Dialysis, Transplantation. 2016;**31**(12):2041-2048. DOI: 10.1093/ndt/gfw074

[112] Chan HW, Clayton PA, McDonald SP, Agar JW, Jose MD. Risk factors for dialysis withdrawal: An analysis of the Australia and New Zealand Dialysis and Transplant (ANZDATA) Registry, 1999-2008. Clinical Journal of the American Society of Nephrology. 2012;**7**(5):775-781. DOI: 10.2215/CJN.07420711

[113] Van Oevelen M, Abrahams AC, Bos WJ, Hoekstra T, Hemmelder MH, Ten Dam M, et al. Dialysis withdrawal in the Netherlands between 2000 and 2019: Time trends, risk factors and Centre variation. Nephrology, Dialysis, Transplantation. 2021;**36**(11):2112-2119. DOI: 10.1093/ndt/gfab244

[114] Chen JH, Lim WH, Howson P. Changing landscape of dialysis withdrawal in patients with kidney failure: Implications for clinical practice. Nephrology. 2022;**27**(7):551-565. DOI: 10.1111/nep.14032

[115] Chen JC, Thorsteinsdottir B, Vaughan LE, Feely MA, Albright RC, Onuigbo M, et al. End of life, withdrawal, and palliative care utilization among patients receiving maintenance hemodialysis therapy. Clinical Journal of the American Society of Nephrology. 2018;**13**(8):1172-1179. DOI: 10.2215/CJN.00590118

[116] Gessert CE, Haller IV, Johnson BP. Regional variation in care at the end of life: Discontinuation of dialysis. BMC Geriatrics. 2013;**13**(1):1. DOI: 10.1186/1471-2318-13-39

[117] Ko GJ, Obi Y, Chang TI, Soohoo M, Eriguchi R, Choi SJ, et al. Factors associated with withdrawal from dialysis therapy in incident hemodialysis patients aged 80 years or older. Journal of the American Medical Directors Association. 2019;**20**(6):743-750. DOI: 10.1016/j.jamda.2018.11.030

[118] Wetmore JB, Yan H, Hu Y, Gilbertson DT, Liu J. Factors associated with withdrawal from maintenance dialysis: A case-control analysis. American Journal of Kidney Diseases. 2018;**71**(6):831-841. DOI: 10.1053/j.ajkd.2017.10.025

[119] McDade-Montez EA, Christensen AJ, Cvengros JA, Lawton WJ. The role of depression symptoms in dialysis withdrawal. Health Psychology. 2006;**25**(2):198. DOI: 10.1037/0278-6133.25.2.198

[120] Davison SN, Jhangri GS. The impact of chronic pain on depression, sleep, and the desire to withdraw from dialysis in hemodialysis patients. Journal of Pain and Symptom Management. 2005;**30**(5):465-473. DOI: 10.1016/j.jpainsymman.2005.05.013

[121] Germain MJ, Cohen LM, Davison SN. Withholding and withdrawal from dialysis: What we know about how our patients die. In: Seminars in Dialysis 2007. Oxford, UK: Blackwell Publishing Ltd

Chapter 9

The Dialyzer as the Last Line of Protection against Endotoxins

Michael Hulko, Werner Beck, Ilona Koch, Rose Speidel and Bernd Krause

Abstract

When dialysis fluid is contaminated with endotoxins, the dialyzer membrane is often referred to as the last line of protection to prevent endotoxins from entering the patient's blood. However, a quantifiable requirement for this endotoxin retention property of the membrane has not yet been defined. The ANSI/AAMI/ISO 23500 standard series provides the framework for the microbiological quality of dialysis water, concentrates, and dialysis fluid, and defines the limit value for the non-pyrogenic endotoxin dose. After defining the boundary conditions of the endotoxin loading of the membrane by dialysis fluid and the patient's non-pyrogenic endotoxin dose, quantifiable requirements for the endotoxin retention properties of a membrane, expressed as a dimensionless logarithmic retention value (LRV), were developed in this work. Based on standard dialysis fluid quality, the LRV should minimally be two for a protein-coated membrane after contact with patient blood and minimally be one for a protein-free pristine membrane during online priming before contact with patient blood. This work also presents the critical factors for endotoxin retention tests and shows that the defined LRV values are reached by membranes in modern dialyzers.

Keywords: dialysis, endotoxins, water quality requirements, membranes, endotoxin retention, pyrogenicity

1. Introduction

In hemodialysis treatment of end-stage renal disease, the patient's blood is separated from dialysis fluid by a semipermeable membrane in the dialyzer. In cases of microbiological contamination of dialysis fluid, it contains pyrogenic substances, such as endotoxins, which would cause fever in the patient if they entered the patient's blood. However, the permeability of the membrane for endotoxins is limited. Therefore, the dialyzer membrane is often called the last line of protection against endotoxins when the microbiological quality of dialysis fluids is discussed. The simplicity of this visualization makes it easy to believe that the underlying concept would have been understood. However, comprehensive and quantitative evaluations and specific definitions of this concept are missing or remain vague. Different situations during a dialysis treatment need to be evaluated in a differentiated manner to account for specific contamination levels, membrane conditions, and fluid flow circumstances. Especially, trends of using online prepared fluid during online priming, online bolus, and online rinse-back need to be examined, since that fluid is filtered across the dialyzer membrane before it is infused into the patient. A verifiable quantitative requirement for the dialyzer membrane to serve as the last line of protection against endotoxins has not yet been defined. This work develops a proposal of how such a requirement could look like.

2. What are endotoxins and can endotoxin retention requirements be inferred from other dialyzer properties?

Endotoxins are mainly lipopolysaccharides (LPS) originating as fragments of bacterial cell membranes. The dominant bacterial source is gram-negative bacteria, which possess an LPS-rich outer membrane. A chemical feature of LPS is their amphiphilic character, which means the molecules combine hydrophilic and hydrophobic parts. This amphiphilic character enables the LPS to form supramolecular structures and biological entities, such as micelles, vesicles, or cell membranes. In those structures, the hydrophobic lipid parts bind together to avoid interaction with water while the hydrophilic polysaccharide parts are exposed to the hydrophilic aqueous environment. This chemical behavior takes place in dialysis fluid and aqueous solutions, in general. More on endotoxins can be found in work done by Williams [1] and Bishop [2].

Dialyzers are primarily designed to remove water and uremic toxins from a patient's blood, and design specifications typically address those requirements. Chemically, uremic toxins are distinctly different from LPS molecules. Uremic toxins are small molecules or proteins that accumulate in the patient's blood when kidney function is impaired. Uremic toxins, even though diverse in chemical nature, are commonly water-soluble in most cases; therefore, do not form larger, aggregated structures in blood plasma water. Water-insoluble uremic toxins bind to albumin, which makes them water-soluble in the albumin-bound form, and they are then called protein-bound uremic toxins.

Dialyzer specifications, such as clearance, sieving coefficient, or ultrafiltration coefficient, as defined and required by technical standards, such as ISO 8637-1 [3], specify the ability to remove water or uremic toxins. Due to the distinct differences in chemical nature and chemical environment of LPS vs. uremic toxins, endotoxin retention properties cannot be simply inferred from specifications describing uremic toxin removal but rather need to be described and investigated in their specific way.

3. How can endotoxin retention properties be characterized and measured?

To measure endotoxin retention properties of a membrane, the concentrations on both sides of the membrane need to be put into relation. The dimensionless ratio of concentrations on the feed side and the filtrate side of the membrane is a practicable relation. Since feed and filtrate concentration typically differ by a few orders of magnitude, it is convenient to transform the ratio as a decadic logarithm into a more practical dimension called logarithmic retention value (LRV).

$$LRV = 10\log\frac{C(Feed)}{C(Filtrate)} \quad (1)$$

It is important to understand that the LRV is not a universally constant intrinsic property of the membrane but rather depends on the conditions under which it has been measured. For a meaningful interpretation of the LRV, it is critical that experimental conditions under which the LRV was measured match the context in which the LRV is to be applied. The fundamental experimental parameters that need to be taken into account are:

- *The concentration of endotoxin on the feed side*. The LRV is a dimensionless number and could be measured in theory at any level of endotoxin concentration. However, the formation of supramolecular structures by LPS depends on the LPS concentration. Since the specific nature of the supramolecular structure may impact the retention properties, and the absolute endotoxin concentration needs to be considered.

- *The concentration of endotoxin on the filtrate side*: In cases of strong LPS retention by a membrane, the concentration on the filtrate side might drop below a detectable concentration level. In such cases, the concentration cannot be assumed as zero. A practical approach for such results is to calculate the LRV using the lower detection limit of the applied assay and report LRV as > the obtained number.

- *Fluid flow conditions*: The transport of solutes across a membrane follows two different mass transport mechanisms: diffusion and convection. Especially, in cross-flow filtration settings, the filtration fraction must be defined carefully because the filtered fluid determines the amount of LPS convectively transported toward the membrane. The fluid flow direction must also be considered. When testing endotoxin retention in the dialysis fluid, the relevant flow direction is from dialysate to the blood compartment, which is the opposite of the ultrafiltration flow direction in hemodialysis.

- *Total endotoxin amount*: The total amount of endotoxins in the feed solution is calculated by multiplying endotoxin concentration with a fluid volume of the feed solution. It plays a role because the mechanism of endotoxin retention by a dialyzer membrane cannot be unambiguously and uniformly described for every membrane. The retention mechanism is likely based on two effects: one is size exclusion of larger LPS aggregates, and the other one is adsorption of LPS molecules by either hydrophobic interaction between the hydrophobic part of the LPS molecule and hydrophobic patches of the membrane or by electrostatic interaction between the negatively charged part of LPS and positive charges of the membrane. Total endotoxin amounts in a test should not be chosen too low and potential saturation of adsorption sites needs to be taken into account.

- *The electrolyte composition of the test fluid*: LPS molecules carry negative charges from phosphate groups in the molecule. These negative charges lead to attractive or repulsive electrostatic forces and impact the formation of supramolecular structures. Especially, double-charged ions, such as Ca^{2+} or Mg^{2+}, in the test fluid can shield the charges in the LPS molecules and influence the formation of the supramolecular structures and LPS retention by the membrane.

- *The temperature of the test fluid*: The temperature of the test fluid affects the formation of supramolecular LPS structures and has a strong impact on diffusion rates.

- *The bacterial source from which the LPS in the test was prepared*: LPS molecules are not uniform, they contain a variable polysaccharide chain, which can differ between bacterial species. This may impact the formation of supramolecular structures and affect how LPS are retained by membranes. What guiding principle can be used to select the bacterial source of LPS? One approach is to select the bacteria species, that is, the most abundant type in microbial contamination. In microbiological studies of dialysis fluid quality [4, 5], the water-borne *Pseudomonas aeruginosa* was the most abundant type of bacteria species found in the dialysis fluid. In cases where the Limulus amebocyte lysate (LAL) assay is used, the selection of LPS can be guided by considering pyrogenic potency. Pyrogenic potency can be measured by testing in rabbits. To avoid animal testing, the LAL assay can be used instead, and manufacturers of the assays match the assay response to a specific LPS preparation using the pyrogenic potency of the rabbit test. An LPS preparation with particular potency in LAL assays can be obtained for LPS, for example, by *Escherichia coli* strains.

- *Absence or presence of a protein layer on the membrane*: In experimental studies, it was observed that a protein layer on the membrane, which forms after the initial contact of the membrane with protein-rich fluids, such as blood plasma, changes endotoxin retention properties compared to a protein-free pristine membrane [6, 7]. Proteins on the membrane are likely to impact pores size, and may also affect surface chemistry, which would account for a modified LPS adsorption to the membrane.

4. Which factors determine endotoxin concentration in dialysis fluid?

The current requirements of dialysis fluid are set out in the ANSI/AAMI/ISO 23500 standards series on the preparation and quality management of fluids for hemodialysis and related therapies. There are two potential sources of endotoxins, water and concentrates, and there is the option to use ultrafilters for endotoxin removal. The water system provides water to the monitor in accordance with the provisions of ANSI/AAMI/ISO 23500-3 (formerly ISO 13959) [8], which defines maximum endotoxin concentration as 0.25 EU/ml for water for dialysis. Concentrates to prepare dialysis fluid to follow the provisions of ANSI/AAMI/ISO 23500-4 (formerly ISO 13958) [9]. Endotoxin concentrations in concentrates must be at a level that allows the preparation of standard dialysis fluid with a maximum of 0.5 EU/ml from concentrate and water for dialysis. The maximum endotoxin concentration for standard dialysis fluid is governed by ANSI/AAMI/ISO 23500-5 (formerly ISO 11663) [10]. If an ultrafilter is used to filtrate the prepared dialysis fluid, ultrapure dialysis fluid can be prepared with a maximum allowed endotoxin concentration of 0.03 EU/ml.

In this work, the assumption is made that dialysis fluid of at least standard dialysis fluid quality per ANSI/AAMI/ISO 23500-5 [10] is provided by the dialysis monitor, and maximum endotoxin concentration is at 0.5 EU/ml even if no ultrafilter is used or in case of failure of the ultrafilter.

5. What is the total endotoxin amount the dialyzer membrane can be exposed to on its dialysate side?

The total endotoxin amount the dialyzer membrane can be exposed to depends on two variables: endotoxin concentration and fluid volume passing or crossing the membrane. In the section above, the assumption of a maximum endotoxin concentration of 0.5 EU/ml was made, because standard dialysis fluid quality per ANSI/AAMI/ISO 23500-5 [10] was assumed in any case. In order to consider the fluid volume passing through or crossing a dialyzer membrane as well as the resulting total amount of endotoxins, various phases and situations during a dialysis treatment need to be differentiated: priming, treatment, bolus, and rinse-back. In the following considerations, only configurations in which online prepared fluid is infused into the patient by crossing the dialyzer membrane are included. Configurations using saline bags or online prepared fluid bypassing the dialyzer membrane are excluded in this work because the dialyzer membrane does not act as a last endotoxin barrier in such situations. Relevant configurations, where the dialyzer acts as the last line of protection against endotoxins are:

- *Online priming with dialysate infusion*: Online priming is used to rinse and fill the dialyzer with online-prepared dialysis fluid. The volume for filling and rinsing is assumed to be up to 3 L. During online priming, the protein-free pristine dialyzer membrane can be exposed to a maximum endotoxin amount of 3000 ml × 0.5 EU/ml = 1500 EU. However, the largest portion of the priming fluid will be discarded, and the patient will not be exposed to the complete priming volume. In cases of "wet" patient connection, (i.e., arterial and venous access are connected simultaneously) the fluid contained within the blood side of the extracorporeal circuit is infused into the patient, which is typically not more than 500 ml. For example, the blood compartment volume of a Polyflux 210 H dialyzer is 125 ml [11], and the fill volume of a single-needle blood line BL 40 SN is 279 ml [12], which sums up to 404 ml.

- *Online bolus with fluid infusion*: Online bolus is used to infuse a specific amount of fluid into the patient, for example, for blood pressure stabilization. Bolus volume can be assumed to be not more than 500 ml per hour. The total maximum endotoxin amount that a protein-coated membrane can be exposed to is 500 ml × 0.5 EU/ml = 250 EU for standard dialysis fluid.

- *Backfiltration and backdiffusion* are physical effects produced by the pressure conditions of the fluidic circuit and the hydraulic permeability of the membrane. The amount of backfiltration is hard to measure or calculate and difficult to predict. It has been calculated and experimentally measured to be in the range of 30–50 ml/min [13] and can be assumed to not exceed 100 ml/min at which dialysis fluid is filtered from dialysate to the blood side of the dialyzer. As a worst-case estimate the maximum endotoxin amount passing the membrane during dialysis treatment can be estimated irrespective of the amount of backfiltration by the total amount of dialysis fluid passing through the dialyzer. Assuming a maximum dialysate flow rate of 800 ml/min of standard quality dialysis fluid with 0.5 EU/ml, the dialyzer would be exposed to a total amount of 800 ml/min × 60 min × 0.5 EU/ml = 24000 EU per hour. If the blood flow rate is lower than the dialysate flow rate, the LPS transfer is physically limited by the blood flow rate, irrespective of whether diffusion or convection is the dominant mass transfer mechanism. Assuming a maximum blood flow rate of 600 ml/min, the maximum amount of endotoxins that could pass through the dialyzer membrane is 600/800 x 24000 EU = 18000 EU per hour.

- *Online rinse-back with fluid infusion*: Rinse-back is the reinfusion of the blood in the blood compartment of the extracorporeal circuit to the patient after treatment. The volume of rinse-back is limited by the volume of the blood pathway of the extracorporeal circuit and can be assumed to be not more than 500 ml. The total maximum endotoxin amount that the protein-coated membrane may be exposed to by rinse-back fluid with standard dialysis fluid quality is 500 ml × 0.5 EU/ml = 250 EU.

6. How much endotoxin could a patient tolerate without developing a pyrogenic reaction?

Various endotoxin dose limits have been developed to prevent pyrogenic reactions during and after medical treatments. The European Pharmacopeia [14] defines a limit of 5 EU/kg body weight per hour for intravenously administered drugs, which is also referenced in ISO 23500-1 [15] as the minimum dose that produces fever and is therefore applied in this work to develop a requirement for the endotoxin retention properties of the dialyzer membrane as the last line of protection against endotoxins. During a 1-hour dialysis session, the upper limit of the endotoxin dose for a patient of 50 kg body weight would be 5 EU/kg/h × 50 kg × 1 h = 250 EU. The body weight was taken from ICH Q3(R8) Guideline [16], which defines 50 kg as "relatively low body weight," to allow some extra safety margin.

7. How much endotoxin must a dialyzer be able to retain?

Two boundary conditions were defined in the previous sections: the endotoxin load on the dialysate side and the non-pyrogenic dose on the blood side. The dialyzer membrane must reduce the endotoxin load on the dialysate side to a non-pyrogenic level on the blood side. With the help of these two boundary conditions, a minimum LRV can be calculated for a dialysis membrane. Since protein-free pristine membranes are different from protein-coated membranes, two requirements can be developed for either case. In the first step, the requirement for a protein-coated membrane will be developed. In the second step, the requirement for the pristine membrane is derived. In the following calculations, the use of standard dialysis fluid will be assumed as worst-case, and the accumulated effects of online bolus, backfiltration/backdiffusion, and online rinse-back are concentrated into 1-hour treatment.

Figure 1 shows the dose calculation for the 1-hour treatment case using standard dialysis fluid of 0.5 EU/ml. Fluid volumes for online bolus and rinse-back are assumed to be 500 ml each. The volume assumed for backfiltration or backdiffusion was derived from a blood flow rate of 600 ml/min being the limiting factor for endotoxin transfer irrespective of the mass transport mechanism; therefore, the volume is 600 ml/min × 60 min = 36 L. The endotoxin amount at each step is calculated as 0.5 EU/ml × fluid volume. This results in 250 EU, 18000 EU, and 250 EU for online bolus, backfiltration/backdiffusion, and online rinse-back, respectively, producing a total of 18500 EU in 1 hour. The minimum LRV (rounded up to 1 significant digit) for the protein-coated membrane to reduce 18500 EU below 250 EU is LRV 2. The dose threshold of 250 EU was calculated using the limits of 5 EU/kg/hour for a 50 kg person as 5 EU/kg/hour x 50 kg × 1 hour = 250 EU. A protein-coated membrane with an LRV of 2 reduces the endotoxin load of 18500 EU on the dialysate side to 185 EU on the blood side.

Figure 2 shows in summarized form the dose calculation when combining the 1-hour treatment case as described above with the online-priming situation with a pristine

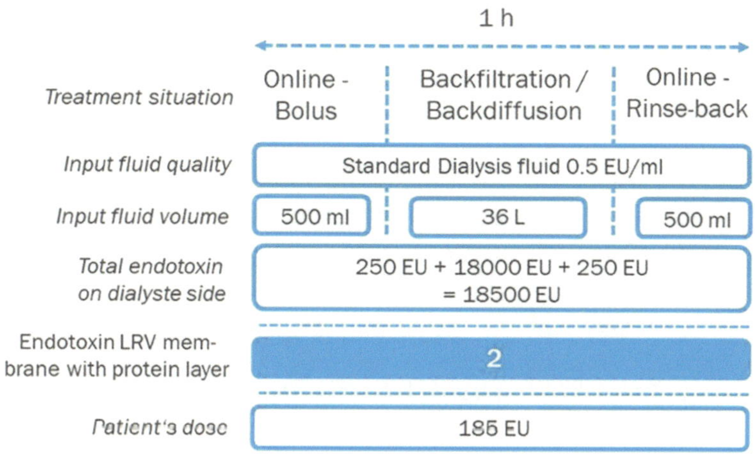

Figure 1.
Calculation of endotoxin load on the feed side, LRV, and endotoxin dose on the filtrate (patient) side for treatment cases, where a protein-coated membrane, reduces the transfer of endotoxins from the standard dialysis fluid.

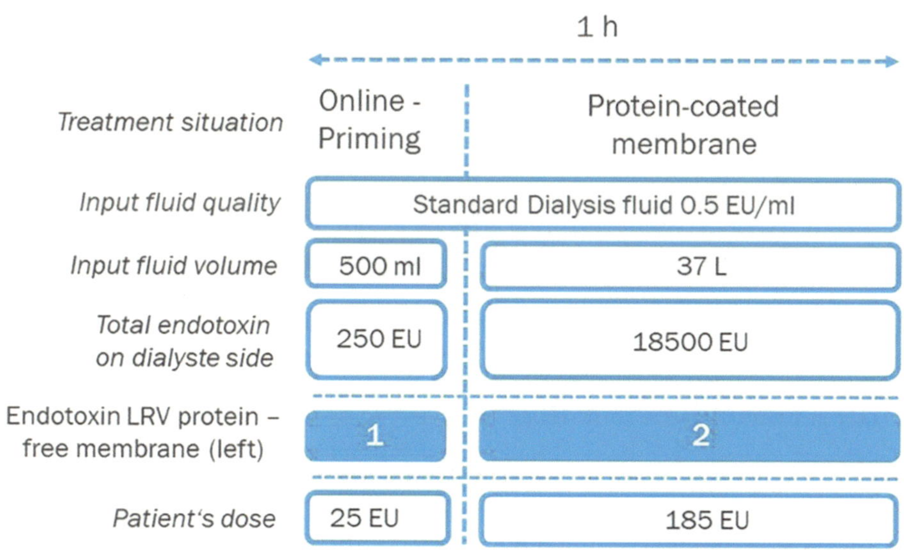

Figure 2.
Calculation of endotoxin load on the feed side, LRV, and endotoxin dose on the filtrate (patient) side for treatment cases, where a protein-coated membrane (right side) and a pristine membrane (left side), reduces the transfer of endotoxins from the standard dialysis fluid.

membrane. The volume of online-priming fluid infused into the patient was assumed to be 500 ml. The endotoxin amount of online priming calculates as 0.5 EU/ml x 500 ml = 250 EU. The dose threshold of 65 EU for online priming can be calculated as the total dose threshold of 250 EU (calculated with the limit of 5 EU/kg/hour for a 50 kg person) minus 185 EU covering online bolus, backfiltration/backdiffusion, and online rinse-back. The minimum LRV (rounded to one significant digit) for the pristine membrane to reduce 250 EU below 65 EU is LRV 1. A pristine membrane with an LRV of 1 reduces the endotoxin load of 250 EU on the dialysate side to 25 EU on the blood side.

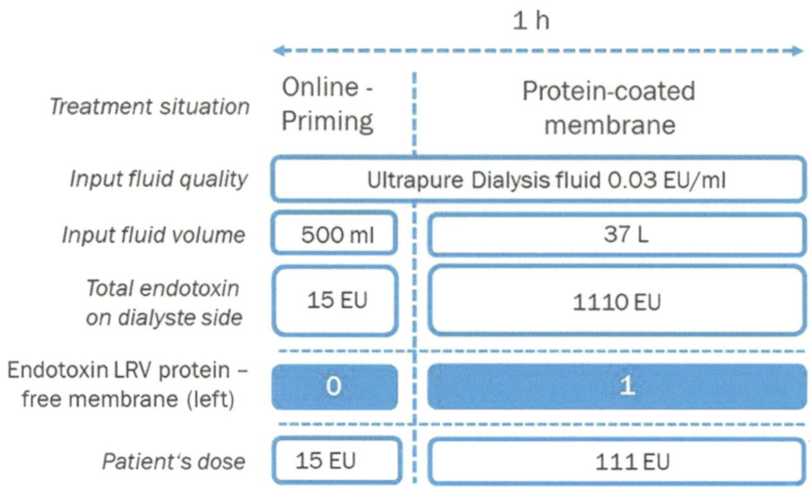

Figure 3.
Calculation of endotoxin load on the feed side, LRV, and endotoxin dose on the filtrate (patient) side for treatment cases, where a protein-coated membrane (right side) and a pristine membrane (left side), reduces the transfer of endotoxins from ultrapure dialysis fluid.

Figure 3 shows a dose calculation for a 1-hour treatment case analogous to the calculations shown in **Figure 2**. The only difference is that the use of ultrapure dialysis fluid of 0.03 EU/ml was assumed instead of standard dialysis fluid. The minimum LRV of the protein-coated membrane would need to be LRV 1 in order to reduce 1110 EU to 111 EU. The pristine membrane would not need to have endotoxin retention properties at all during online priming. The total endotoxin dose of 126 EU (111 EU + 15 EU= 126 EU) would be below the endotoxin dose limit of 250 EU (5 EU/kg/hour for a 50 kg patient).

8. What should a requirement for the endotoxin barrier property of a dialyzer membrane look like?

The calculations above show different endotoxin retention requirements for standard dialysis fluid and ultrapure dialysis fluid. Although the use of ultrapure dialysis fluid is recommended and it is not mandatory, and in the case of the absence or failure of an ultrafilter, only standard fluid quality can be assumed. Consequently, a requirement must orient itself to the use of standard dialysis fluid quality.

For standard dialysis fluid, a dialyzer membrane must have a minimum endotoxin retention capacity measured as an LRV of 2 after exposure to blood plasma and the formation of a protein layer, and it must have a minimum LRV of 1 in its protein-free pristine form.

Is this a realistic requirement for current, state-of-the-art dialyzer membranes? The LRVs of dialyzer membranes with a protein layer are well documented under treatment conditions. Polyflux L (low flux), Revaclear (high flux), and Theranova (medium cut-off) dialyzers were tested in various experimental configurations using mixed filtrates of *Pseudomonas aeruginosa* and *Pelomononas saccharophila* [17], lysates of *Pseudomonas aeruginosa* and isolated LPS from *Escherichia coli* [18]. In all cases, the LRV was above 2 [18]. Experimental data in the perspective of this work is not available for pristine membranes. An experimental study is described in the sections below to provide data to answer the question if the minimum LRV requirement of LRV 1 is realistic for state-of-the-art dialyzer membranes before protein contact.

9. Experimental study to determine endotoxin LRV of a protein-free membrane under online-priming test conditions

Test articles were high flux dialyzers Polyflux 210H and Revaclear 500, as well as medium cut-off dialyzer Theranova 500. The products were taken from regular manufacturing with standard sterilization and within their specified shelf-life. For each type of dialyzer, the test items were taken from three separate production lots. Revaclear 500, Theranova 500, and Polyflux 210H are the products with the largest membrane area of their respective product family. In this study, the product with the largest membrane area in each product family was chosen because it provides the largest interface between the dialysate and the blood side compartment. An experimental pre-study under online-priming test conditions did not indicate an impact by the membrane area between 1.4 m^2 and 2.1 m^2 on endotoxin retention properties and, if adsorptive retention was assumed, a saturation of adsorptive capacity was not observed for smaller and larger membrane areas. Under this presumption, the items selected for testing in this study can be considered to be representative under online-priming conditions for versions with smaller membrane area down to 1.4 m^2 in their respective product family.

The sample number was defined to be six (6). The sample number definition was not based on a formal statistical approach. Previous studies had shown 95% confidence intervals within a range of ± 10% of the mean LRV for a similar experimental design using six samples.

The test system had two parts. The first part comprised sample generation, and the second part the sample analysis.

Sample generation was done in a benchtop experiment of filtration (**Figure 4**). Fluid from a challenge solution made of endotoxin-contaminated bicarbonate-based dialysis fluid was pumped by a peristaltic pump across a dialyzer membrane. The fluid flow direction in the dialyzer was from dialysate to blood side. The filtrate was collected on the blood side for subsequent analysis.

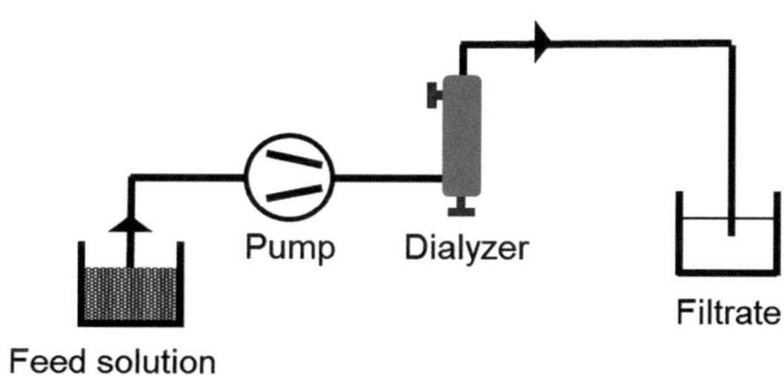

Figure 4.
Schematic drawing of the filtration setup. A feed solution containing a defined amount of endotoxin is pumped through the dialyzer using a peristaltic pump. Flow direction is from dialysate to blood compartment. Unused ports of the dialyzer were blocked. The filtrate was collected on the blood side.

Test setting	Set value	Justification
Composition of feed fluid.	Bicarbonate-based dialysis fluid prepared from dialysis concentrate D200 (MTN Neubrandenburg, Code 20000060401) Acid concentrate D204 (MTN Neubrandenburg, 20400100001, 1.75 mM Ca^{2+}. 0.5 mM Mg^{2+} in final fluid). Reverse osmosis water. Before adding endotoxins, the dialysis fluid was sterile filtered using a U9000 plus Ultrafilter (Baxter) and checked for pH 7.1–7.5	Bicarbonate dialysis fluid is a state-of-the-art dialysis fluid.
Bacterial endotoxin from two different sources.	1. *Escherichia coli* strain O55:B5 (Lonza, Code 00193783) 2. *Pseudomonas aeruginosa* (Sigma-Aldrich, Code L9143)	*Escherichia coli* O55:B5 is an endotoxin, which is traceable to a defined reference standard material; therefore, suitable to provide accurate endotoxin concentrations [1]. *Pseudomonas aeruginosa* is a common water-borne organism and can be found in dialysis fluid; therefore, represents clinical conditions [4, 5].
Bacterial endotoxin concentration in feed fluid.	The bacterial endotoxin concentration must be > 0.5 EU/ml; the targeted set value was 2 EU/ml.	0.5 EU/ml is the maximum allowed endotoxin concentration in standard dialysis fluid according to ANSI/AAMI/ ISO 23500-5 [10] and therefore the minimum concentration in this study to represent worst-case clinical conditions.
Volume of feed solution	3000 ml[1]	3000 ml was assumed as maximum rinse volume and is considered as worst-case in this study because it results in the largest possible endotoxin amount.
Fluid temperature	37°C +/− 2°C	37°C +/- 2°C was assumed as clinically relevant temperature range of the priming fluid.
Fluid flow rate	200 ml/min +/− 10%	200 ml/min was assumed as maximum priming flow rate. No impact by flow rate between 100–500 ml/min was observed in a feasibility study. Nevertheless, 200 ml/min is considered to be worst-case, as it results in a minimum time that the endotoxin interacts with the membrane, which minimizes potential interactions; +/− 10% was assumed typical flow accuracy.
Sampling at two sampling points at end of sample generation.	1. Sample of about 2 ml was taken from the filtrate at the end of filtration. 2. Sample of about 1 ml was taken from the feed solution at the end of the filtration.	Sample at the end of filtration represents the dialysis fluid that remains in the extracorporeal circuit and could be infused into the patient in clinical practice. A sample from the challenge solution was taken for LRV calculation.

[1]*Volumetric measurement accuracy range within the accuracy range of the scale of suitable measurement cylinders.*

Table 1.
Sample generation test settings and justification.

Filter type	Sample #	LRV (*P. aer*)	LRV (*E. coli*)
Revaclear 500	1	2.6	>2.8
	2	>2.5	2.6
	3	>2.6	>2.6
	4	>2.4	>2.5
	5	>2.7	>2.7
	6	>2.5	>2.6
Polyflux 210H	1	>2.5	>2.6
	2	>2.6	>2.6
	3	>2.3	>2.6
	4	>2.0	>2.5
	5	>2.2	>2.7
	6	>2.4	>2.6
Theranova 500	1	2.5	>2.8
	2	2.3	2.5
	3	>2.7	>2.6
	4	>2.7	>2.5
	5	2.3	>2.7
	6	>2.4	>2.6

Table 2.
Results of the experimental study. LRV was measured using the protein-free pristine membrane under online-priming conditions. LRV is shown for Pseudomonas aeruginosa (P. aer) and Escherichia coli (E. coli). When LRV was calculated using the lower limit of detection of the LAL assay (0.005 EU/ml) values are shown as "> ."

Table 1 identifies and specifies the critical settings and provides justification for the selected value.

The challenge solution was filtered directly through the dry dialyzer to simulate the clinical priming process.

A portion of each feed sample was diluted 10x with bicarbonate-based dialysis fluid. A diluted sample was needed in certain cases to bring the endotoxin concentration within the working range of the endotoxin assay. The endotoxin concentration was determined using Limulus amebocyte lysate (LAL) assay in accordance with the manufacturer's instruction and validated using local work instruction

The results obtained are shown in **Table 2**.

In conclusion, all dialyzers tested met the proposed LRV requirement of a minimal LRV of 1, for both types of endotoxin, LPS from *Pseudomonas aeruginosa* and *Escherichia coli* under conditions of online priming with dialysate infusion.

10. Discussion and conclusion

This work aimed to develop and propose a measurable requirement to define the retention properties of the dialyzer being the last line of protection against endotoxins potentially present in the dialysis fluid. By setting out the boundary conditions of the endotoxin load on the feed side and the tolerable endotoxin dose on the patient side, a requirement could be defined. The requirement employed the concept of the dimensionless logarithmic retention value (LRV). Since protein-free pristine membranes and protein-coated membranes show different endotoxin retention properties, two requirements were developed, one for each case. The requirement for protein-coated membranes is a minimum LRV of 2, and the requirement for protein-free pristine membranes is a minimum LRV of 1. These requirements are based on the assumption that standard dialysis fluid per ISO 23500-5 [10] can be provided at any time by controlling the water system, the concentrates, and potential ultrafilters in the mixing unit (dialysis monitor). The development of the requirements considered various treatment conditions, where fluid can cross the dialyzer membrane from dialysate to blood side or endotoxins could pass by diffusion from dialysis fluid into the patient's blood. During the development of the requirements, worst-case considerations were employed when specific values were selected from a potential range. Maximum endotoxin concentrations and fluid volumes were assumed—to represent the highest possible endotoxin load—while on the patient side a relatively low body weight was selected. When backfiltration and backdiffusion during a dialysis treatment were taken into account, the hypothetical transfer of all endotoxins across the membrane was considered, which is probably an overestimation to some degree, because a large amount of endotoxins will probably just bypass the membrane in the dialysis fluid stream due to diffusion rate limitations. The proposed endotoxin requirements are realistic for state-of-the-art dialyzers; reference literature supported this for protein-coated membranes [17, 18], and experimental data were presented for protein-free pristine membranes. Even though standard dialysis fluid can be used to perform dialysis therapy according to ISO 23500-1 [15], it also stated that "standard dialysis fluid shall be regarded as the minimum acceptable quality. Ultrapure dialysis fluid is a step forward in improving biocompatibility, reducing inflammation, and preventing dialysis-related complications."

Acknowledgements

The authors thank the cross-functional team members who supported this work. The financial contribution was supported by Baxter International Inc.

Conflict of interest

All authors are employed by Gambro Dialysatoren GmbH (Affiliate of Baxter International Inc.).

Legal disclaimer

The manufacturer of the tested dialyzers does not extend any representation or warranty (expressed or implied) regarding the dialyzers that go beyond the respective instructions for use or product labels of the dialyzers. The manufacturer of the dialyzers shall in no event be held liable for the suitability of the dialyzers beyond the label information.

Author details

Michael Hulko*, Werner Beck, Ilona Koch, Rose Speidel and Bernd Krause
Gambro Dialysatoren GmbH (Affiliate of Baxter International Inc.), Hechingen, Germany

*Address all correspondence to: michael_hulko@baxter.com

References

[1] Williams KL. Endotoxins: Pyrogens, LAL Testing and Depyrogenation (Drugs and the Pharmaceutical Sciences, # 167). 3rd ed. Boca Raton, USA: Taylor & Francis Inc

[2] Bishop RE. Fundamentals of endotoxin structure and function. Contributions to Microbiology. 2005;**12**:1-27

[3] ISO 8637-1. Extracorporeal Systems for Blood Purification — Part 1: Haemodialysers, Haemodiafilters, Haemofilters and Haemoconcentrators. Geneva, Switzerland. 2017

[4] Vanholder R et al. Endotoxin transfer through dialysis membranes: Small- versus large-pore membranes. Nephrology, Dialysis, Transplantation. 1992;7(4):333-339

[5] Lonnemann G. Assessment of the quality of dialysate. Nephrology, Dialysis, Transplantation. 1998;**13** (Suppl. 5):17-20

[6] Lonnemann G et al. The role of plasma coating on the permeation of cytokine-inducing substances through dialyser membranes. Nephrology, Dialysis, Transplantation. 1995;**10**(2):207-211

[7] Schindler R et al. Blood components influence cytokine induction by bacterial substances. Blood Purification. 2001;**19**(4):380-387

[8] ANSI/AAMI/ISO 23500-3. Preparation and Quality Management of Fluids for Haemodialysis and Related Therapies—Part 3: Water for Haemodialysis and Related Therapies. Arlington, USA. 2019

[9] ANSI/AAMI/ISO 23500-4. Preparation and Quality Management of Fluids for Haemodialysis and Related Therapies—Part 4: Concentrates for Haemodialysis and Related Therapies. Arlington, USA. 2019

[10] ANSI/AAMI/ISO 23500-5. Preparation and Quality Management of Fluids for Haemodialysis and Related Therapies—Part 5: Quality of Dialysis Fluid for Haemodialysis and Related Therapies. Arlington, USA. 2019

[11] Baxter Polyflux H Dialzer Brochure (GLBL/MG3/18-0020e - 2019

[12] Baxter Novaline bloodline tubing system Brochure (GBU-RC60-210001 v5.0 – February 2022)

[13] Lorenzin A et al. Quantification of internal filtration in hollow fiber hemodialyzers with medium cut-off membrane. Blood Purification. 2018;**46**:196-204

[14] European Pharmacopoeia 5.0 2.6.14. Bacterial Endotoxins. Strasbourg: Council of Europe

[15] ANSI/AAMI/ISO 23500-1. Preparation and Quality Management of Fluids for Haemodialysis and Related Therapies—Part 1: General Requirements. Arlington, USA. 2019

[16] ICH Harmonised Guideline - Impurities: Guideline for Residual Solvents Q3C(R8) Current Step 4 version dated 22 April 2021

[17] Schepers E et al. Assessment of the association between increasing membrane pore size and endotoxin permeability using a novel experimental dialysis simulation set-up. BMC Nephrology. 2018;**19**(1):1. DOI: 10.1186/s12882-017-0808-y

[18] Hulko M et al. Pyrogen retention: Comparison of the novel medium cut-off (MCO) membrane with other dialyser membranes. Scientific Reports. 2019;**9**(1):6791. DOI: 10.1038/s41598-019-43161-2

Chapter 10

Expanded Hemodialysis Therapy: From the Rational to the Delivery

Nadia Kabbali and Basmat Amal Chouhani

Abstract

Expanded hemodialysis therapy is a new concept in blood purification technology using a specific membrane with a steep sieving curve characterized by medium membrane cutoff and high retention onset values that are close to but lower than those of albumin. Expanded hemodialysis therapy thereby targets an important pathophysiologic link to many of the sequelae of end-stage renal disease, by improving the clearance of medium to larger-size solutes. The significant internal filtration achieved in these hemodialyzers provides a remarkable convective clearance of medium to high solutes. This therapy does not need specific software or additional complex technology, making its application possible in every setting once the quality of the dialysis fluid is guaranteed to ensure the safe conduct of the dialysis session. The present chapter reviews the rationale for expanded hemodialysis therapy, the potential benefits, and the considerations for prescription and delivery.

Keywords: expanded hemodialysis, membrane cutoff, retention onset, internal filtration, medium molecular weight solutes

1. Introduction

In 2010, more than 2 million individuals worldwide were receiving maintenance dialysis, and this number was expected to increase to 5.4 million by 2030 [1]. Despite improvements in technology and medical care, the mortality rate of patients on maintenance dialysis remains high, with 55% dying within 5 years of initiating dialysis therapy [2]. It has even been shown that the survival in maintenance dialysis patients was lower than that for patients with several types of cancer [3].

This mortality is largely related to the accumulation of uremic toxins. The existence of an interaction between uremic toxins, inflammation and/or oxidative stress, and cardiovascular mortality is well reported in the various epidemiological studies. In accordance with the European Uremic Toxins Work Group (EUTox) database, there are currently more than 153 uremic solutes listed, and that number should increase over time [4].

According to the molecular weight of these uremic toxins, they are divided into six classes, including small water-soluble molecules (<500 Da), protein-bound uremic toxins (PBUTs; mostly <500 Da), small-middle molecules (0.5–15 kDa), medium-middle molecules (15–25 kDa), large-middle molecules (25–58 kDa), and large molecules (>58 kDa) [5]. Complications, such as anemia, neuropathies, osteodystrophy, dialysis-related amyloidosis, accelerated atherosclerosis, and cardiovascular complications, have been correlated with uremic toxins in the molecular range of 5–50 kDa [6].

Originally, membranes for hemodialysis were designed to remove small solutes, such as urea and creatinine. Since then, technological progress has continued to develop to improve the clearance of uremic toxins. The advent of ultrafiltration control systems led to the development and use of high-flux (HF) membranes that allowed improved middle molecule removal. Further evolution in technology led to the development of a new class of membranes referred to as super-flux or high cutoff (HCO), with albumin loss representing a limitation to their practical application. Hemodiafiltration (HDF) at high volumes (>23 L/1.73 m2/session) has produced some results on middle molecules and clinical outcomes, although complex hardware and high blood flows are required. A new class of membranes has recently been developed with characteristics allowing high clearances of solutes in a wide spectrum of molecular weights without significant loss of albumin. These membranes originally defined as "medium cutoff" are probably better classified as "high retention onset" and have introduced a new concept of hemodialysis called "expanded hemodialysis" (HDx). It is a simple dialysis technique, requiring no sophisticated equipment or special training for nurses, making its application possible in every setting once the quality of the dialysis fluid is guaranteed to ensure the safe conduct of the dialysis session.

In this chapter, we describe the characteristics of the medium cutoff membranes, their potential benefits, and considerations for the prescription and delivery of HDx.

2. Medium cutoff (MCO) membranes characteristics

2.1 Radius and distribution of membrane pores

Dialyzers' surface properties are crucial factors in evaluating the membrane performance. The morphological characteristics, such as mean pore size, pore size distribution, surface porosity, and pore tortuosity, influence the molecular weight removal spectrum and membrane clearance. For the MCO membrane, the size of the pores is intermediate between those of the HF and HCO membranes [7]. The MCO membrane has an effective pore radius of 3.0–3.5 nm after contact with blood, allowing for the removal of an expanded range of uremic toxins [8]. The distribution of the pores in dialysis membranes is not uniform. The more the membrane pore size distribution curves are deviated to the right, the better the removal of large middle molecules, but the risk of albumin loss is higher, it is the case with HCO membranes [9]. To improve the clearance of large middle molecules, while avoiding the loss of albumin, the distribution of the pore sizes has had to be "tightened." This is the principle used in MCO membranes.

In addition to the tight distribution of pores, there are two major differences between the MCO membrane and with HF dialyzer: first, the wall thickness is decreased from 50 μm to 35 μm, which allows a shorter diffusion path, second, the diameter of hollow fibers inside MCO membranes is reduced from the standard 200 μm to 180 μm, to improve convection and internal filtration (see internal filtration chapter below).

2.2 Sieving curves

One of the main characteristics of a dialysis membrane is its permeability in terms of sieving capacity. The sieving curve shows a progressive reduction of the observed values for solute sieving as the solute molecular weight increases. Molecular weight cutoff (MWCO) is defined as the lowest molecular weight (in daltons) at which greater than 90% of a solute with a known molecular weight is retained by the membrane (sieving = 0.1). On the other side of the sieving curve, the molecular weight at which 10% of the solute is retained (sieving = 0.9) defines the retention onset of the membrane (MWRO). A classification scheme was proposed in which the MWCO and the MWRO are utilized in combination to define different dialyzer classes. As the separation between MWRO and MWCO decreases, the profile of the curve becomes steeper, resulting in increased removal of large uremic toxins and decreased loss of albumin [10]. Based on this concept of selectivity of the sieving coefficient, we can now differentiate the different membranes. MCO membrane, although presenting a similar MWRO to the HCO membrane, displays a completely different behavior. While MWRO for the HF membrane is in the range of 1200 Da (vitamin B12), MWRO for the MCO membrane is in the range of 12,000 Da (β-2 microglobulin). On the other side, when comparing MCO and HCO membranes, we see that these two membranes will have the same performance when extracting middle molecules, such as β-2 microglobulin, with a high MWRO for the two membranes, however, the MCO membrane has a much lower MWCO for albumin, thus making it possible to limit the leaks of albumin. For this reason, the MCO membranes have also been defined as high retention onset membranes (HRO), with the aim of optimizing clearances of medium to large MW solutes while avoiding significant albumin loss [11].

2.3 Internal filtration

Clearance of middle molecules cannot be improved by diffusive phenomena alone; convective clearance must also be optimized. Let us remember that convective clearance (K) results from the product of the UF rate (Qf) and sieving (S) of the selected molecule (K = Qf x S). Because the sieving of the selected molecule is low, the only way to increase K is to increase Qf. The on-line hemodiafiltration (OL-HDF) has made high convection rates possible thanks to the combined pre- and post-dilution configuration, but complex hardware and high blood flows are required. Due to the specific internal properties of the MCO membrane, HDx with MCO membranes represents a simpler way to improve convective clearance, with no need for fluid substitution. The ultrafiltration control system of regular hemodialysis machines provides the exact amount of net filtration required for the scheduled weight loss of dialysis patients. In OL-HDF, large amounts of ultrafiltration (UF) are achieved with high transmembrane pressure (TMP) and then replaced in the venous line after multiple steps of filtration of fresh dialysate. In HDx, the convection flow is maintained in the first part of the MCO membrane, based on excessive ultrafiltration due to the mentioned characteristics of this membrane, but it is compensated by the mechanism of internal filtration inside the filter, which takes place at about the terminal part of this membrane, and is considered as replacement fluids to the ultrafiltration [6].

The remarkable amount of convection in the proximal part is resulting from an increased end-to-end pressure drop. Internal filtration compensates for the excessive filtration rate in the distal part [12]. Thus, the convective transport of MCO membranes increases by a large margin along the length of the fibers, which makes it possible to remove large molecules with low diffusion coefficients. Indeed, to improve solute transport and avoid protein stagnation at the blood membrane interface, the diameter of hollow fibers inside MCO membranes is reduced from the standard 200 μm to 180 μm [13], which increases the rate of wall shear and blood flow velocity

[14]. Reducing the diameter and thickness of the membrane can increase internal convection by up to 30%. The combination of hydraulic permeability and geometric structure of the fibers enhances the process of internal filtration in MCO membranes [15]. MCO membranes are thus characterized by higher permeability than classic high-flux membranes. Blood flow ≥300 mL/min and dialysate flow ≥500 mL/min is sufficient to achieve optimal clearance in the system [6, 11].

3. Potential benefits of MCO membranes in HDx

3.1 Removal of ß2-microglobulin (B2M)

ß2-microglobulin is a 99 amino acid protein produced by all nucleated cells with the exception of red blood cells, it has a molecular weight of 11.8 k Daltons. It plays an important role in the immune system; it is involved in the defense against bacterial and viral infections as well as in the prevention of cancerous cells [16]. B2M accumulation in dialysis can lead to its aggregation into amyloid fibers that deposit in joint spaces causing a dialysis-related amyloidosis, resulting in carpal tunnel syndrome, arthropathy, and organ deposition of amyloid proteins [17]. It can also cause inflammation and immune dysfunction. B2M accretion has been associated with a decrease in residual kidney function [18] and an increased risk of all-cause, cardiovascular and infectious deaths [19–20]. Serum B2M remains positively associated with mortality, in a study of 23,976 patients, conducted by the Dialysis Outcomes and Practice Patterns Study (DOPPS) over a period of 10 years [17].

Convective techniques, including HDF and HF dialysis, provide better removal of middle molecules. In addition, several randomized controlled studies suggest that HF dialyzers are more effective in removing B2M than low flux membranes. Regarding HDx, studies have shown that HDx with MCO membranes results in a greater reduction ratio of a broad range of molecules, including B2M compared to HF membranes [8, 20–23]. There are several factors that can affect the clearance of B2M [8], in the study conducted by Lim [24], the reduction ratio achieved was slightly lower, and the B2M clearance was not significantly different, which was probably due to a low blood flow rate. B2M levels were found to be more important than initial levels even after one year of HDX.

Another factor that may influence the inability to remove the B2M is the rebound phenomenon, probably secondary to resistance due to a massive transfer between different body compartments that limits the clearance of B2M [25], leading sometimes to an increase in B2M levels even with MCO membranes [26].

3.2 Removal of free light chain (FLC)

Monoclonal free light chains of immunoglobulin kappa or lambda isotype have a molecular weight of 22.5 kDa and 45 kDa, respectively. They are metabolized by the kidney and can be detected in blood or urine. These FLC can polymerize in the form of dimer or multimer and thus reach high molecular weights of up to 900 kilodaltons [8]. Recently, they have been identified as toxic molecules in uremic patients [27]. Serum FLC levels have been shown to be associated with increased mortality in end-stage renal disease [27]. Therefore, FLC could be biomarkers of medium and large molecules that can be eliminated by hemodialysis, especially since their determination is not expensive and are available in most laboratories. In patients with dialysis-dependent myeloma cast nephropathy, early FLC removal by intensive hemodialysis (IHD) with an adsorbent polymethylmethacrylate membrane (IHD-PMMA) combined with chemotherapy was associated with high rates of renal recovery and survival [28]. In a multicenter randomized trial, including 172 hemodialysis patients showed that the reduction ratio of FLC kappa and lambda was significantly higher in the HDx group using Theranova membranes compared to the use of high flux dialysis with Elisio-17H dialyzers after 6 months. This reduction was maintained in HDx until subsequent dialysis sessions [29].

3.3 Chronic inflammation

Chronic inflammation is a major and known complication during the end-stage renal disease. Among others, serum concentration of beta2-microglobulin and inflammatory mediators have been correlated with malnutrition-inflammation-atherosclerosis and formation of amyloid deposits in bone, tendons, and joints [30]. Indeed, oxidative stress results from a disequilibrium between pre-oxidative and anti-oxidative products, several molecules of high and medium molecular weight have increased levels, particularly the pro-inflammatory cytokines interleukins 1β, 6, 18, and TNF-α with prolongation of their half-life due to the uremic state. The clinical consequences are malnutrition, increased cardiovascular risk, erythropoietin resistance, and increased all-cause mortality [31].

Studies have suggested a better removal of pro-inflammatory proteins with MCO membranes and HDx. In a study conducted on patients with acute kidney injury and sepsis suspected of having high cytokine levels, the use of MCO membrane in continuous veno-venous hemodialysis (CVVHD) had a modest clearance of most cytokines and demonstrated small to no adsorptive capacity despite a decline in plasma cytokine concentrations [32] while in the randomized crossover trial of 48 hemodialysis patients, comparing MCO dialysis to HF dialysis for 12 weeks, the authors showed a considerable reduction in the expression of cytokines -RNAm of IL2 and TNFα, in circulating leucocytes when using MCO, compared to HF dialyzers. This study showed that MCO could significantly reduce inflammatory mediators in the first weeks. This difference was absent when the study was extended to 12 weeks. There was a decrease in the initial albumin concentration with stabilization thereafter [33].

In a prospective study [34], the MCO dialysis membranes had a favorable outcome on inflammation with a decrease in C-reactive protein levels when compared to low-flow dialysis and high-flux membranes, without any effect on oxidative stress markers (paraoxonase-1, ischemia-modified albumin, total Thiol, disulfide bond, and native Thiol). In addition, in Cozzolino et al. study, there was a 50% reduction in infection rate that requires admission and systemic antibiotics in patients treated with expanded hemodialysis enabled by the medium cutoff membrane [35].

3.4 Cardiovascular parameters

It is well established that cardiovascular damage is the primary cause of morbidity and mortality in end-stage renal disease. Several factors are involved or may contribute to their aggravation (increased phospho-calcium product with vascular calcification, anemia, inflammation, and oxidative stress). Uremic toxins can induce platelet activation and aggregation, leading to the development of thrombi [36].

In a clinical trial comparing the reduction of vascular smooth muscle cell calcifications *in vitro* by MCO and HF membranes, vascular calcifications were significantly reduced *in vitro* by 24% after 4 weeks and by 33% after 12 weeks in the MCO group compared to the HF group. The concentration of calcification-associated proteins (Matrix Gla, osteopontin (OPN) and growth differentiation factor 15 (GDF-15)) was higher after incubation with HF compared to MCO. This suggests that expanded hemodialysis reduces the potential for calcifications in dialysis serum *in vitro*; these results remain to be proven *in vivo* [37]. Ciceri et al. performed a prospective, controlled, cross-over study, comparing HDx and conventional hemodialysis to analyze the pro-calcifying serum of uremic patients. Uremic serum of HDx-treated patients induced less vascular smooth muscle cells (VSMC) necrosis compared with uremic serum of HD patients. However, no differences were found between dialytic treatments in the serum potential to induce apoptosis and to modulate the expression of a panel of genes involved in VSMC simil-osteoblastic differentiation [38].

Regarding the clinical impact of HDx on cardiovascular parameters, a prospective randomized controlled trial enrolled 80 patients with HDX and HDF online. The first criterion evaluated was the changes in brachial-ankle pulse wave velocity, which did not differ between the HDX group with MCO and the HDF group. Echocardiographic parameters and cardiovascular mortality were comparable in the two groups with a tendency to increase the coronary artery calcium score in HDx [36]. HDx with MCO membranes could be a good alternative when online-HDF is not available.

3.5 Removal of proteins binding to uremic toxins (PBUT)

Despite their small molecular weight, proteins bound to albumin are difficult to remove by conventional methods. Among these molecules homocysteine, which is three to four times higher in dialysis patients, can cause inflammation, endothelial lesions, and cardiovascular damage [39]. Other small molecules, such as 3-Carboxy4-methyl-5-propyl-2-furanpropionate (MPF), tryptophan and some of its metabolites, such as indoxyl sulfate (IS), 3 indol acetic acid, kynurenine, and p-cresulfate (p-CS), bind to albumin making their removal difficult. Theoretically, a decrease in albumin would allow the elimination of these PBUTs, but studies conducted to compare this clearance between HDx and conventional HD showed contradictory results regarding the elimination of these molecules [40]. A sub-study of the REMOVAL-HD trial, enlisting 89 participants, found no significant changes in total or free levels of IS or p-CS after 12 or 24 weeks of MCO membrane use compared to baseline, as no significant albumin loss was observed in this study. Whereas an open-label, controlled, cross-over study comparing HDx and conventional HD found a significant decrease in IS and other metabolites in the HDx group [38]. Further long-term, randomized studies are needed to prove whether PBUTs clearance by HDx is superior to other techniques and to evaluate its clinical impact.

3.6 Quality of life

The evaluation of health-related quality of life (QOL) in end-stage renal disease became more and more important. Patients on dialysis suffer from symptoms, such as fatigue, cramps, loss of appetite, and pruritus [41]. Those signs are mostly related to the accumulation of uremic toxins, anemia, and cardiovascular complications, which altered mental and physical health. A decrease in QOL is also associated with an increase in mortality [42].

Several studies aimed to compare the use of HDx with conventional hemodialysis or HDF in improving QOL parameters, using several scores (LEVIL, KDQOL -SF 36, PROM POS-S Renal Symptom questionnaire and the "Recovery time from last dialysis session) [43, 44]. The major items assessed were dialysis symptom index, restless legs syndrome, sleep, energy, and well-being. In a prospective multicenter observational study of the COREXH registry, 992 patients were switched from HF to HDx for one year. The results showed that the items' symptoms, effects of kidney disease, and burden of kidney disease, improved as well as restless leg syndrome, which decreased significantly over a 12-month monitoring period [45]. Multiple studies [24, 46] showed an upgrade in QOL in patients on HDx compared to HDF or conventional HD. Bolton et al., when switching from regular high-flux dialysis membrane to medium cutoff (MCO) membrane, and evaluating different symptoms burden by the POS-S Renal total symptom score, showed a decrease at 6 months. The fatigue and lack of energy improved constantly; the percentage of participants scoring its impact as "severe" decreased from 28% at baseline to 16% at 12 months [44]. Other studies using the KDQol-36 and the Edmonton symptom assessment system revised (ESAS-r), did not demonstrate any effect of HDx on QOL [29, 47]. Studies were conducted to evaluate biomarkers for the best use of the distinctive features and benefits of HDF, α 1-MG is one biomarker that could evaluate this removal performance. The authors concluded that hemodiafilter should provide an α 1-MG removal rate of 35%. An improvement in clinical manifestations can be expected by doing so, and it increases patients' QOL [48].

The HDx with MCO membranes can improve the QOL of patients. The use of this technique may be of use in the targeted selection of patients and assist in monitoring response. The study's results are encouraging and suggest the use of HDx even in patients who cannot benefit from convective techniques because of vascular access or intolerance to high volumes of exchange [49].

3.7 Safety concerns

3.7.1 Albumin loss

HDx allows the removal of large molecules (>45 k daltons), including albumin, due to its large pore size distribution [39]. In the studies that evaluated albumin removal by HDx, there was a controversy between those showing a significant decrease versus those where the level of albumin remained the same. Even when the decrease was significant, there were no clinical signs of hypoalbuminemia, some patients reported a better appetite after switching to the HDx therapy [29, 45]. This is probably due to better removal of leptin, obsestatin, and acyl ghrelin associated with a drop in appetite among dialysis patients [50].

In the large observational study from the COREXH registry, the observed variability from baseline and maximum average change in mean serum albumin levels were − 1.8% and − 3.5%, respectively. No adverse events were related to the MCO membrane [51].

On the other hand, a slight decrease in serum albumin might be beneficial for dialysis patients. HDx might induce a moderate removal of PBUTs, oxidized albumin, and carbamylated albumin along with the serum albumin loss [51].

3.7.2 Pyrogene retention

The larger pore sizes of MCO membranes have raised concerns about the potential for increased membrane permeability to pyrogens including endotoxins and other bacterial contaminants that could be present in the dialysis fluid, which can contribute to the pathological features of uremia in patients receiving dialysis. Hulko et al. tested the capacity of low-fux, high-fux, MCO, and HCO dialyzer membranes with different pore sizes to prevent pyrogens crossing from dialysate to the blood side in a closed-loop test system, differentiating among lipopolysaccharides, peptidoglycans, and bacterial DNA using a toll-like receptor assay. Levels of lipopolysaccharides, peptidoglycans, and bacterial DNA in the blood-side samples were too low to identify potential differences in pyrogen permeability among the membranes [52].

In another study by Schepers et al., four dialysis membranes of comparable composition but with different pore sizes were tested for their permeability for endotoxins by exposing them during a 1 h *in vitro* dialysis session to dialysate contaminated with filtrates of two water-borne bacteria, *Pseudomonas aeruginosa* and *Pelomonas* saccharophila, at an endotoxin challenge at least four times the upper limit of endotoxin load (2 EU/ml) when using standard dialysis fluid. For the tested membranes, there was a nonsignificant difference in the number of the polyvinylpyrrolidone solutions, which contained a detectable amount of endotoxin after repetitive circulation through the dialyzer, be it close to the detection limit in the majority of cases [53].

These results suggest that MCO membranes are suitable for hemodialysis using ISO standard dialysis fluid quality [54], and retain endotoxins at a similar level as other membranes.

3.7.3 Effects on medication clearance

The question that comes to mind is whether the increased pore size in MCO membranes affects the retention of commonly used medications or coagulation factors in dialysis patients. Very few clinical studies have addressed this issue [55].

Using an *in vitro* model, removing erythropoietin, heparin, insulin, and several coagulation factors with HDx was comparable with HF and HDF therapy, suggesting that it is not necessary to change the medication dosing or anticoagulation protocols for dialysis patients receiving HDx therapy with MCO membranes. In the study published by Allawati et al., vancomycin clearance was higher in the MCO group compared to high-flux the group, but it was not statistically significant [56].

3.7.4 Routine use evaluation of MCO membranes

In the study by Florens et al., the authors evaluated the first routine use of HDx therapy in real-life conditions. Eighteen centers participated, and nurses and nephrologists answered by filling in a score regarding the use of MCO membranes. The assessment was related to packaging, priming, and rinsing of the dialyzers. Overall HDx therapy was easy to use in routine, and no adverse events were reported. However, nurses experienced some issues concerning poor de-aeration and the need for more anticoagulation. These problems could be prevented by training the medical staff [50].

4. For whom and how to make the prescription?

In view of the potential beneficial clinical effects associated with the use of HDx, most patients on chronic hemodialysis would be potential candidates for HDx treatment, especially since, to our knowledge, there is currently no specific contraindication to the use of MCO membranes in patients on chronic hemodialysis. That said, some criteria can help us to choose the patients to start with and gain experience in HDx therapy.

As HDx would optimize the clearance of middle molecules, it would ideally be prescribed in patients who have the greatest retention of large middle molecules and those who would have the greatest benefit from increased removal of these molecules. Among these patients, mention may be made of anuric patients, since serum concentrations of middle-molecules are closely correlated with residual renal function, patients with a long-expected lifespan, without kidney transplant project, patients with persistent hyperphosphatemia, and patients with chronic inflammation, erythropoietin resistance, secondary immunodeficiency, and cardiovascular disease [30, 57]. Moreover, there are some promising applications in which HDx could have an interest: pruritus, post-HD asthenia, anorexia, restless legs syndrome, myeloma, and rhabdomyolysis [50].

Compared to the OL-HDF, the HDx would be useful when an adequate convective volume (23 L) cannot be reached (elevated hemoglobin, suboptimal blood flow...), or when the OL-HDF needs to be suspended (dialysis without anticoagulation, one needle puncture, safety reasons) [7]. HDx is a simple dialysis technique, requiring no sophisticated equipment or special training for nurses. It can be delivered with any standard hemodialysis monitor. As described above, blood flow around 300 mL/min and dialysate flow around 500 mL/min is sufficient to achieve optimal clearance, superior to HF hemodialysis and comparable to or even exceeding HDF [13]. HDx therapy requires no specific or intensified clinical monitoring. However, as with all filters with internal filtration, the quality of dialysis fluid remains a sine qua non condition to ensure the safe conduct of the dialysis session. The manufacturer recommends that the MCO membrane should not be used in convective strategies most likely due to the potential risk of significant albumin loss [30]. Thus, especially in patients who were in HDF, or when using monitors that can perform HDF, care should be taken to verify the selected treatment mode, and switch the treatment mode to hemodialysis if not.

Another factor that should probably be considered is the length of the session. In comparison to small water-soluble solutes, the clearance of middle-molecules is affected more by the inter-compartment transfer from extra to intravascular compartments during dialysis [30]. So, it would make sense that, at least in dialysis settings where time is flexible, such as home hemodialysis, MCO membranes could be used for long or more frequent dialysis treatments to increase middle-molecule removal.

5. Conclusion

Despite advances in hemodialysis-related technologies, there was no clear progress in terms of mortality benefit and clinical outcome. The ability to remove medium-high uremic toxins could provide a potential advantage. A number of dialyzers were developed over time, from low flow membranes to high flow dialyzers, the clearance of these molecules is still limited. The most recent and promising advance in the field of hemodialysis is represented by the development of medium-cutoff, high-retention-onset membranes. The combination of conventional hemodialysis and MCO membranes define expanded hemodialysis, this innovation in the field of dialysis allows diffusion and convection in a hollow fiber dialyzer. This gives it the capacity to purify middle and large molecules without the need for large convective volumes and without a significant albumin loss. Its simple setup and application offer the possibility to use it even in patients with suboptimal vascular access or even with an indwelling catheter. Larger studies would be needed to further quantify any beneficial effects of HDx on major clinical events. Morbidity and mortality clinical studies are needed to demonstrate at least the non-inferiority of HDx over OL-HDF.

Conflict of interest

The authors declare no conflict of interest.

Author details

Nadia Kabbali[1,2]* and Basmat Amal Chouhani[1,2]

1 Department of Nephrology, Dialysis, and Transplantation, Hassan II University Hospital, Fez, Morocco

2 Laboratory of Epidemiology and Health Science Research (ERESS), Faculty of Medicine, Sidi-Mohammed-Ben-Abdellah University, Fez, Morocco

*Address all correspondence to: kabbalinadia@gmail.com

References

[1] Liyanage T, Ninomiya T, Jha V, et al. Worldwide access to treatment for end-stage kidney disease: A systematic review. Lancet. 2015;**385**(9981):1975-1982

[2] Canadian Institute for Health Information. Canadian Organ Replacement Register Annual Report: Treatment of End-Stage Organ Failure in Canada, 2003 to 2012. Ottawa, ON, Canada: CIHI; 2014

[3] Naylor KL, Kim SJ, McArthur E, Garg AX, McCallum MK, Knoll GA. Mortality in incident maintenance dialysis patients versus incident solid organ cancer patients: A population-based cohort. American Journal of Kidney Diseases. 2019;**73**(6):765-776

[4] Vanholder R, Glorieux G, De Smet R, Lameire N. European uremic toxin work group: New insights in uremic toxins. Kidney International. Supplement. 2003;**63**:S6-S10

[5] Rosner MH, Reis T, Husain-Syed F, Vanholder R, Hutchison C, Stenvinkel P, et al. Classification of uremic toxins and their role in kidney failure. Clinical Journal of the American Society of Nephrology. 2021;**16**:1918-1928

[6] Ronco C, Marchionna N, Brendolan A, Neri M, Lorenzin A, Martínez Rueda AJ. Expanded haemodialysis: From operational mechanism to clinical results. Nephrology, Dialysis, Transplantation. 2018;**33**(suppl_3):iii41-iii47

[7] Perez-Garcia R, Alcazar-Arroyo R, de Sequera-Ortiz P. What is the role of expanded hemodialysis in renal replacement therapy in 2020? Nefrologia (Engl Ed). May-Jun 2021;**41**(3):227-236

[8] Kirsch AH, Lyko R, Nilsson L-G, Beck W, Amdahl M, Lechner P, et al. Performance of hemodialysis with novel medium cut-off dialyzers. Nephrology, Dialysis, Transplantation. 2017;**32**:165-172

[9] Wolley M, Jardine M, Hutchison CA. Exploring the clinical relevance of providing increased removal of large middle molecules. Clinical Journal of the American Society of Nephrology. 2018;**13**:805-814

[10] Ronco C, Clark WR. Haemodialysis membranes. Nature Reviews. Nephrology. 2018;**14**(6):394-410

[11] Ronco C. The rise of expanded hemodialysis. Blood Purification. 2017;**44**:I-VIII

[12] Macias N, Vega A, Abad S, Aragoncillo I, Maria Garcia-Prieto A, Santos A, et al. Middle molecule elimination in expanded haemodialysis: Only convective transport? Clinical Kidney Journal. 2019;**12**:447-455

[13] Ronco C, La Manna G. Expanded hemodialysis: A new therapy for a new class of membranes. Contributions to Nephrology. 2017;**190**:124-133

[14] Ronco C, Brendolan A, Lupi A, Metry G, Levin NW. Effects of a reduced inner diameter of hollow fibers in hemodialyzers. Kidney International. 2000;**58**:809-817

[15] Fiore GB, Ronco C. Principles and practice of internal hemodiafiltration. Contributions to Nephrology. 2007;**158**:177-184

[16] Miyata T, Jadoul M, Kurokawa K, van Ypersele de Strihou C. b2 microglobulin

in renal disease. Journal of American Society and Nephrology. 1998;**9**:1723-1735

[17] Eiichiro K, Daniel M, Bieber B. Beta-2 microglobulin and all-cause mortality in the era of high-flux hemodialysis: Results from the dialysis outcomes and practice patterns study. Clinical Kidney Journal. 2021;**14**(5):1436-1442. DOI: 10.1093/ckj/sfaa155

[18] Argyropoulos CP, Chen SS, Ng YH, et al. Rediscovering beta-2 microglobulin as a biomarker across the spectrum of kidney diseases. Frontiers in Medicine (Lausanne). 2017;**4**:73

[19] Cheung AK, Greene T, Leypoldt JK, et al. Association between serum 2-microglobulin level and infectious mortality in hemodialysis patients. Clinical Journal of the American Society of Nephrology. 2008;**3**:69-77

[20] Watanabe Y, Kawanishi H, Suzuki K, et al. "Maintenance hemodialysis: Hemodialysis prescriptions" guideline working group, Japanese Society for Dialysis Therapy. Japanese society for dialysis therapy clinical guideline for "maintenance hemodialysis: Hemodialysis prescriptions". Therapeutic Apheresis and Dialysis. 2015;**19**:67-92

[21] Nistor I, Palmer SC, Craig JC, Saglimbene V, Vecchio M, Covic A, et al. Convective versus diffusive dialysis therapies for chronic kidney failure: An updated systematic review of randomized controlled trials. American Journal of Kidney Diseases. 2014;**63**(6):954-967 Epub 2014 Jan 14

[22] Yang,H, Ke, G, Liao,Y, et al Efficacy of medium cut-off dialyzers and comparison with high-flux dialyzers in patients on maintenance hemodialysis: A systematic review and meta-analysis. Therapeutic Apheresis and Dialysis 2022;**26**(4):756-768

[23] Hung YH, Lai TS, Belmouaz M, Tu YC, Lai CF, Lin SL, et al. Effects of medium cut-off polyarylethersulfone and polyvinylpyrrolidone blend membrane dialyzers in hemodialysis patients: A systematic review and meta-analysis of randomized controlled trials. Membranes (Basel). 20 Apr 2022;**12**(5):443

[24] Lim J-H, Park Y, Yook J-M, Choi S-Y, Jung H-Y, Choi J-Y, et al. Randomized controlled trial of medium cut-off versus high-flux dialyzers on quality of life outcomes in maintenance hemodialysis patients. Scientific Reports. 2020;**10**:7780

[25] Ward RA, Greene T, Hartmann B, Samtleben W. Resistance to intercompartmental mass transfer limits beta2-microglobulin removal by post-dilution hemodiafiltration. Kidney International. 2006;**69**:1431-1437

[26] Cho N-J, Park S, Islam I, Song H-Y, Lee EY, Gil H-W. Long-term effect of medium cut-off dialyzer on middle uremic toxins and cell-free hemoglobin. PLoS One. 2019;**14**:e0220448

[27] Fraser SD, Fenton A, Harris S, Shardlow A, Liabeuf S, Massy ZA, et al. The Association of Serum Free Light Chains with mortality and progression to end-stage renal disease in chronic kidney disease: Systematic review and individual patient data meta-analysis. Mayo Clinic Proceedings. 2017;**92**:1671-1681

[28] Sens F, Chaintreuil D, Jolivot A, Guebre-Egziabher F, Robinson P, Karlin L, et al. Effectiveness of IHD with adsorptive PMMA membrane in myeloma cast nephropathy: A cohort study. American Journal of Nephrology. 2017;**46**(5):355-363

[29] Weiner DE, Falzon L, Skoufos L, Bernardo A, Beck W, Xiao M, et al.

Efficacy and safety of expanded hemodialysis with the Theranova 400 dialyzer. Clinical Journal of the American Society of Nephrology. 2020;**15**:1310-1319

[30] Hutchison CA, Wolley M. The rationale for expanded hemodialysis therapy (HDx). In: Ronco C, editor. Expanded Hemodialysis – Innovative Clinical Approach in Dialysis. Vol. 191. Basel, Karger: Contrib Nephrol; 2017. pp. 142-152

[31] Tenvinkel P et al. IL-10, IL-6, and TNF-alpha: Central factors in the altered cytokine network of uremia – The good, the bad, and the ugly. Kidney International. 2005;**67**:1216-1233

[32] Lumlertgul N, Hall A, Camporota L, Crichton S, Osterman MC. Clearance of infammatory cytokines in patients with septic acute kidney injury during renal replacement therapy using the EMiC2 flter (Clic-AKI study). Lumlertgul et al. Critical Care. 2021;**25**:39

[33] Zickler D, Schindler R, Willy K, Martus P, Pawlak M, Storr M, et al. Medium cut-off (mco) membranes reduce inflammation in chronic dialysis patients—A randomized controlled clinical trial. PLoS One. 2017;**12**:e0169024

[34] Yeter HH, Korucu B, Akcay OF, Derici K, Derici U, Arinsoy T. Effects of medium cut-off dialysis membranes on inflammation and oxidative stress in patients on maintenance hemodialysis. International Urology and Nephrology. 2020;**52**:1779-1789

[35] Cozzolino M, Magagnoli L, Ciceri P, et al. Effects of a medium cut-off (TheranovaVR) dialyser on haemodialysis patients: A prospective, cross-over study. Clinical Kidney Journal. 2021;**14**(1):382-389

[36] Lee Y, Jang M-J, Jeon J, Lee JE, Huh W, Choi BS, et al. Cardiovascular risk comparison between expanded hemodialysis using theranova and online hemodiafiltration (CARTOON): A multicenter randomized controlled trial. Scientific Reports. 2021;**11**:10807

[37] Willy K, Girndt M, Voelkl J, Fiedler R, Martus P, Storr M, et al. Expanded hemodialysis therapy of chronic haemodialysis patients prevents calcification and apoptosis of vascular smooth muscle cells in vitro. Blood Purification. 2018;**45**:131-138

[38] Ciceri P, Tettamanti G, Galassi A, et al. Pro-calcifying analysis of uraemic serum from patients treated with medium cut-off membrane in a prospective, cross-over study. Clinical Kidney Journal. 2021;**14**(7):1798-1807

[39] Zhang Z, Yang T, Li Y, Li J, Yang Q, Wang L, et al. Effects of expanded hemodialysis with medium cut-off membranes on maintenance hemodialysis patients: Review. Membranes. 2022;**12**(3):253

[40] Jourde-Chiche N, Dou L, Cerini C, Dignat-George F, Brunet P. Vascular incompetence in dialysis patients-protein-bound uremic toxins and endothelial dysfunction. Seminars in Dialysis. 2011;**24**:327-337

[41] Abdel-Kader K, Unruh ML, Weisbord SD. Symptom burden, depression, and quality of life in chronic and end-stage kidney disease. Clinical Journal of the American Society of Nephrology. 2009;**4**:1057-1064

[42] Tsai Y-C, Hung C-C, Hwang S-J, Wang S-L, Hsiao S-M, Lin M-Y, et al. Quality of life predicts risks of end-stage renal disease and mortality in patients with chronic kidney disease.

Nephrology, Dialysis, Transplantation. 2010;**25**:1621-1626

[43] Penny JD, Jarosz P, Salerno FR, Lemoine S, McIntyre CW. Impact of expanded hemodialysis using medium cut-off dialyzer on quality of life: Application of dynamic patient-reported outcome measurement tool. Kidney Medicine. 29 Jul 2021;**3**(6):992-1002.e1

[44] Bolton S, Gair R, Nilsson LG, Matthews M, Stewart L, McCullagh N. Clinical assessment of dialysis recovery time and symptom burden: Impact of switching hemodialysis therapy mode. Patient Related Outcome Measures. 4 Nov 2021;**12**:315-321

[45] Alarcon JC, Bunch A, Ardila F, Zuñiga E, Vesga JI, Rivera A, et al. On behalf of the colombian registry of expanded hemodialysis investigators impact of medium cut-off dialyzers on patient-reported outcomes: COREXH registry. Blood Purification. 2021;**50**:110-118

[46] Reis T, Martino F, Dias P, de Freitas GRR, Filho ERDS, de Azevedo MLC, et al. Removal of middle molecules with medium cutoff dialyzer in patients on short frequent hemodialysis. Hemodialysis International. 2021;**25**:180-187

[47] Krishnasamy R, Hawley CM, Jardine MJ, Roberts MA, Cho Y, Wong M, et al. A trial evaluating mid cut-off value membrane clearance of albumin and light chains in hemodialysis patients: A safety device study. Blood Purification. 2020;**49**:468-478

[48] Sakurai K. Biomarkers for evaluation of clinical outcomes of Hemodiafiltration. Blood Purification. 2013;**35**(suppl. 1):64-68

[49] Gernone G et al. Long-term evaluation of the HDx on dialysis adequacy, anaemia and quality of life. Nephrology, Dialysis, Transplantation. 2020;**35**(Suppl. 3):P1084.5

[50] Florens N, Juillard L. Expanded haemodialysis: News from the field. Nephrology, Dialysis, Transplantation. 2018;**33**(suppl_3):iii48-iii52

[51] Berg AH, Drechsler C, Wenger J, Buccafusca R, Hod T, Kalim S, et al. Carbamylation of serum albumin as a risk factor for mortality in patients with kidney failure. Science Translational Medicine. 2013;**5**:175ra29

[52] Hulko M, Dietrich V, Koch I, et al. Pyrogen retention: Comparison of the novel medium cut-off (MCO) membrane with other dialyser membranes. Scientific Reports. 2019;**9**:6791

[53] Schepers E, Glorieux G, Eloot S, et al. Assessment of the association between increasing membrane pore size and endotoxin permeability using a novel experimental dialysis simulation set-up. BMC Nephrology. 2018;**19**:1

[54] ISO 23500-5:2019. Preparation and Quality Management of Fluids for Haemodialysis and Related Therapies — Part 5: Quality of Dialysis Fluid for Haemodialysis and Related Therapies [Internet]. Available from: https://www.iso.org/standard/67614.html [Accessed: January 9, 2023]

[55] Voigt M, Gebert M, Haug U, Hulko M, Storr M, Boschetti-De-Fierro A, et al. Retention of beneficial molecules and coagulation factors during haemodialysis and haemodiafiltration. Scientific Reports. 2019;**9**:6370

[56] Allawati H, Dallas L, Nair S, Palmer J, Thaikandy S, Hutchison CA. Pharmacokinetic study comparing the clearance of vancomycin during haemodialysis using medium cut-off

membrane (Theranova) and high-flux membranes (Revaclear). Toxins. 2020;**12**:317

[57] Heyne N. Expanded hemodialysis therapy: Prescription and delivery. Contributions to Nephrology. 2017;**191**:153-157

Chapter 11

Anesthetic Management of Surgical Vascular Access for Hemodialysis

Koichiro Nandate

Abstract

Patients with end-stage renal disease (ESRD) have an adjusted all-cause mortality rate significantly higher than the general population. Surgical techniques to establish hemodialysis access are common and increasing in frequency as more and more patients are diagnosed with advanced and end-stage renal disease. The purpose of this review is to focus on the fundamentals of perioperative anesthetic management of a patient who is scheduled for hemodialysis access procedure. This involves not only the choice of anesthesia method but also pre-anesthesia preparation, intraoperative and postoperative management, and the effect of choice of anesthesia on the outcomes.

Keywords: anesthesia, vascular access, hemodialysis, end-stage renal disease, anesthesia management

1. Introduction

1.1 Pre-anesthesia preparation at anesthesia clinic

A comprehensive preoperative evaluation is mandatory for safe and effective anesthesia management since chronic kidney disease (CKD) is an independent risk factor for predicting postoperative death and cardiac events [1]. Therefore, the evaluation should be most efficiently done in a pre-anesthesia clinic. It is essential to identify the comorbidities that are common to patients with chronic or end-stage renal disease, including coronary artery disease and hypertension. Once identified, measures and treatments should be initiated to medically optimize these patients to minimize or eliminate the risk of surgery and anesthesia. Current guidelines recommend checking a baseline electrocardiogram (ECG) in those patients who have cardiovascular risk factors or documented cardiovascular disease [1]. Additionally, the patient should be scheduled to have routine hemodialysis. Ideally, hemodialysis should be done one day prior to the surgery. Basic laboratory tests including a complete blood count and metabolic and coagulation panel may also be considered in pre-anesthesia clinics.

1.2 Same day evaluation

Most procedures done to establish hemodialysis access are outpatient procedures with patients arriving a few hours prior to the planned procedure. The pre-anesthesia evaluation in the preoperative holding area is one of the most important phases in preparing the patient for the administration of anesthesia. The anesthesia team should confirm that the patient's general condition has not changed since they are evaluated in pre-anesthesia clinic. The site of intravenous access and blood pressure measurement must be avoided in the arteriovenous (AV) access arm. Establishing peripheral intravenous access may be challenging, and an ultrasound-guided method may be helpful to identify an appropriate vein. In cases where a patient has an existing indwelling catheter, consideration can be taken to gain access. However, this is generally avoided due to fear of increased infectious complications. Routine airway examination should be done at the same time even if general anesthesia is not planned.

1.3 Special anesthetic considerations: chronic vs end-stage renal disease

For those patients with chronic renal disease but have not yet started hemodialysis. It is important to ask the patients about the volume and regularity of daily urine production with special attention to those who report a recent drop in volume and/or frequency. This may indicate a recent worsening of their renal function, which may necessitate closer attention to potassium changes or fluid management during the procedure. For those patients already on hemodialysis, it is important to establish when the patient underwent hemodialysis last. Ideally, the patient is expected to have hemodialysis 12 to 24 hours prior to the procedure to facilitate their physiologic status to completely or near completely return to normal at the time of anesthetic administration. Additionally, whether the patient has routine hemodialysis regularity or not is also important since a single session of dialysis may not normalize the patient who does not undergo regular hemodialysis, particularly the fluid status. Similarly, it is important to ask if the patient is well tolerated during the last hemodialysis session. If the patient felt uncomfortable during hemodialysis, the session was not completely terminated, or the patient skipped a regular session because of feeling ill, it may indicate other factors that must be seriously considered. These factors, combined with laboratory abnormalities, may necessitate canceling/rescheduling the procedure.

1.4 Which laboratory data are important?

Verification of certain laboratory data is critical to check on the day of the procedure as these patients are subject to day-to-day changes.

1.4.1 Potassium

The serum potassium levels in patients with chronic renal or end-stage renal disease are typically elevated. Hyperkalemia is potentially life-threatening and must not be neglected. There are no "cut off" levels of preoperative potassium levels to consider for canceling the case or proceeding the procedure safely. Therefore, the potassium level used to determine "go or not go" may vary among hospitals. It should be noted that the serum potassium level is closely related to serum pH. Therefore, if the patient is acidotic, re-evaluation of serum potassium level must be considered after serum pH is corrected. In our institution, a potassium level higher than 6.0 mmol/L prompts a discussion between the anesthesia and surgical teams regarding the need for urgent hemodialysis prior to the procedure. One additional consideration is that venous potassium levels can sometimes falsely be higher than arterial levels. Obtaining and checking an arterial blood sample may be useful in confirming the correct true potassium level [2]. Occasionally, patients can have a lower preoperative potassium level (<3.5 mmol/L). Hypokalemia is not as dangerous for patients as hyperkalemia. Therefore, correction is required if it is associated with frequent cardiac arrhythmias or with significant EKG changes such as QT prolongation. It is extremely difficult to correct hypokalemia in a patient with ESRD. Therefore, consultation with a nephrologist or a cardiologist is safer to avoid overcorrection with possible cardiac complications.

1.4.2 Hemoglobin and hematocrit

Patients with chronic or end-stage renal disease are mostly status of "chronic anemia" due to lower erythropoietin activity as well as the effect of uremic toxic metabolites on bone marrow. Anemia does not need to be corrected routinely since it is well tolerated by patients due to the gradual progression of anemia. There are no definite guidelines regarding the hematocrit level below which blood products should be transfused. However, previous studies have reported increased intraoperative complications in patients with end-stage renal disease and preoperative hematocrit levels ranging from 20–26% [3]. Hemodialysis access surgery itself is usually not a procedure with significant surgical blood loss. Therefore, more flexible criteria may be accepted for transfusion. However, transfusion should be considered if the patient is symptomatic or has significant comorbidities such as history of coronary artery disease and/or cerebrovascular disease beyond specific objective criteria of hemoglobin and hematocrit. It should be noted that transfusion of blood products may increase the patient's potassium level [4] as well as induce antibody formation which may decrease a patient's chances of successful renal transplantation in the future [5].

1.4.3 Coagulation panel

Patients with chronic or end-stage renal disease may have coagulopathy due to platelet dysfunction, decreased coagulation factors, and/or fragile capillary vessels. Additionally, if the patients have uncontrolled atrial fibrillation and cerebrovascular and/or peripheral vascular disease, they have chronic anticoagulation treatment such as warfarin and/or antiplatelet therapy such as aspirin or clopidogrel. Patients are usually instructed to temporally hold oral anticoagulants prior to the procedure, but occasionally it is not carried out. In this situation, there may be additional limitations to the surgery or could necessitate canceling/rescheduling the procedure. In the case of a prolonged bleeding time or elevated INR, a regional nerve block may be contraindicated due to risk of bleeding complications with hematoma formation and nerve compression.

2. Choice of anesthesia

After the evaluation of the patient's physical condition, anesthesia method should be decided. Anesthetic options include local anesthetic (LA) infiltration around the operative site provided by the surgical team in combination with monitored anesthesia care and sedation (MAC (Monitored Anesthesia Care)) provided by the anesthesia team, regional anesthesia (RA), and general anesthesia (GA). Choice of anesthesia also depends on the surgical site and the type of surgery. The surgery for vascular access for hemodialysis can essentially be categorized into two basic types such as arteriovenous fistulas (AVF) and arteriovenous grafts (AVG).

For AVF, a fistula is created between an artery and a vein. There are two common sites in the upper extremity where a fistula is created: between the radial artery and cephalic or basilic vein at the wrist and between the brachial artery and cephalic or basilic vein in the upper arm. For AVF created with the basilic vein, transposition of the vein is required, affecting the chosen anesthesia method. Alternatively, AVG is placed using prosthetic material between an artery and vein in the forearm or upper arm. Any of the three options (LA, RA, and GA) are acceptable for both AVF and AVG. However, the patient's medical comorbidities, the anatomic location (wrist/forearm, antecubital fossa, and upper arm), and the surgeon's preference are to be considered when selecting the anesthesia method.

Choice of anesthetic options can be determined based on the anatomic location of surgical incision. LA with MAC can be considered suitable for the procedures performed at the wrist and the antecubital fossa. RA is a viable option for procedures performed at the antecubital fossa and distal upper arm. GA or RA with an interscalene block can be considered when procedures involve the proximal upper arm for AVG and transpositions, which require tunneling.

2.1 Local anesthesia

Infiltration of LA in the surgical field by the surgeon provides stable analgesia with minimal to no hemodynamic and respiratory changes and is, therefore, often used in patients who have severe cardiopulmonary co-morbidities. The specific LA selected depends on the surgeon's preference, but many surgeons prefer 1% lidocaine as the onset is faster compared to others. In some patients experiencing agitation or anxiety during the procedure, LA alone is not well tolerated. This situation should be overcome with additional sedation and/or analgesia such as propofol infusion or fentanyl provided by the anesthesia team. The other problem for LA is the lack of a preventive effect on the spasm of the artery, in contrast to RA and GA. Previous reports have revealed that the use of a brachial plexus block with a supraclavicular approach provided dilatation of both the veins and arteries of the ipsilateral extremity immediately following the block, reduced the incidence of arterial spasm during and after the surgery, and significantly decreased the rate of immediate AVF failure postoperatively when compared to those that were performed with LA [6–8].

2.2 Regional anesthesia

RA of the upper extremity is primarily achieved through a brachial plexus block. RA offers many advantages over other anesthetic methods, including intraoperative hemodynamic stability and good postoperative analgesia. There is also evidence that it improves vascular flow via regional sympathectomy, although evidence of improved graft survival is lacking yet [6–8]. There are several ways to perform a brachial plexus block, including supraclavicular or infraclavicular and axillary approaches. Complications of RA include infection, hematoma, local anesthetic toxicity, and nerve injury. There are also complications that are specific to each approach, such as total spinal anesthesia, Horner syndrome, hemi diaphragmatic paralysis, and pneumothorax during supraclavicular blocks. There is not enough published data, but the use of ultrasound-guided nerve blocks certainly appears to have made these blocks easy and decreased the incidence of complications [9]. It should be noted that following a brachial plexus block supplementation with LA by the surgeon may be required and LA dose calculations are to be kept in mind to avoid local anesthetic toxicity.

2.2.1 Supraclavicular block

The supraclavicular block is performed around the brachial plexus and passes with the subclavian artery, which is an exceptionally good anatomical landmark. The subclavian artery crosses over the first rib between the insertions of the anterior and middle scalene muscles, posterior to the midpoint of the clavicle. A high frequency (10–15 MHz) ultrasound beam due to the superficial location of the brachial plexus at this level should be used to improve the quality of visualization of all structures in this area. The subclavian artery is readily apparent as an anechoic round structure, while the parietal pleura and the first rib can be seen as a linear hyperechoic structure immediately lateral and deep to the subclavian artery. Supraclavicular brachial plexus can be visualized slightly superficial and posterolateral to the subclavian artery. Local anesthetic solution is given over the trunks of the brachial plexus above the formation of musculocutaneous and axillary nerves [10]. The supraclavicular block is preferred in many institutes because the brachial plexus is tightly packed at this level allowing for an intensive block. Also, this block provides adequate anesthesia for the entire arm and allows for surgical site flexibility. The major disadvantage is relatively higher risk for pneumothorax due to its proximity to the pleura, but it can be overcome with use of ultrasound technique. Also, phrenic nerve blockade is likely (reported up to 50% incidence) with this approach and close observation should be performed especially in patients with compromised respiratory function. The supraclavicular block should be avoided in patients who are unable to withstand up to 30% reduction in pulmonary function resulting from ipsilateral phrenic nerve block.

2.2.2 Infraclavicular block

The infraclavicular block is performed around the brachial plexus, which is below the level of the clavicle and in proximity to the coracoid process. Local anesthetic solution is deposited over the cords of the brachial plexus, which lie circumferentially around the artery at this level. This block is indicated for distal arm surgery at the elbow, forearm, and hand. Due to the relatively deep location of the brachial plexus at this level, lower frequency of ultrasound beam (5–12 MHz) is helpful for better tissue visualization, especially in obese patients whose plexus is extremely deep [11]. Maneuvers to decrease the depth of the target may be worth trying for success. Some patients may feel uncomfortable with this block since the needle should penetrate through the thicker muscles such as pectoralis major and minor. The patients may require more sedation, which may be respiratory depression or apnea. It should be noted that supplementation of LA provided by the surgeon, additional sedation, or conversion to general endotracheal anesthesia may be required if additional high surgical approach of forearm is needed. In some institutes, this block is considered as an alternate for supraclavicular when there is a relative contraindication to supra-clavicular block (e.g., subclavian artery pathology or arteriovenous communication around the trunks, which makes it difficult to pass the needle without puncturing the vessels; severe chronic obstructive pulmonary disease).

2.2.3 Axillary block

The axillary block performed under ultrasound guidance is highly recommended and successful. Due to the superficial location of the brachial plexus, high-frequency ultrasound beam (10–15 MHz) can provide an excellent visualization of all structures where local anesthetics are injected. The axillary artery is a very good landmark to find the spot to find location of the median, ulnar, radial, and median nerves. An additional block of the musculocutaneous nerve off the axillary artery is required to achieve complete analgesia for distal arm. However, it should be noted that there are significant variations between the anatomical positions of the nerves relative to the axillary artery [12]. More analgesic effect is achieved by multiple injections rather than a single injection for axillary approach. Retzl and colleagues observed that the position of the nerves relative to the axillary artery at this level changes significantly with application of varying pressures [13].

2.3 General anesthesia

Almost all patients with CKD and ESRD have multiple comorbid risk factors for GA due to the nature of the conditions that led to the renal insufficiency. Previous clinical research has reported that approximately 25% of the patients who undergo renal replacement therapy have ischemic heart disease, 10% have cerebrovascular disease, and 12% have peripheral vascular disease [14]. Therefore, anesthesiologists consider avoiding GA, if possible, but this may not always be feasible for patients with a history of psychological disorders or those who need more complicated procedures, such as an upper arm transposition or AVG, which may not be amenable to RA. Modes of GA delivery include endotracheal tube (GETA) and laryngeal mask (LMA). There are some advantages of GETA over LMA. GETA provides a more secure airway and controls $PaCO_2$ easily. It results in minimal aspiration risk and avoids respiratory acidosis that can contribute to increase the potassium level rapidly. However, usage of LMA does not require muscle relaxants, which can delay emergence from GA at the conclusion of the case.

During anesthesia induction, hemodynamics should be maintained with titrating doses of inductions agents such as propofol and prompt use of narcotics. However, blood pressure tends to decrease significantly after induction due to lower vascular compliance and/or lower cardiac reserve function. In these cases, a bolus or a continuous infusion of vasoactive medications such as ephedrine and phenylephrine intravenously should be initiated at the same time as general anesthesia induction to keep the perfusion pressure adequate. Also, selection for induction drugs such as etomidate or midazolam combined with fentanyl, which do not decrease blood pressure as much as propofol, may be a good idea. As to pain control during the surgery, the use of LA by the surgeon can contribute to reducing the intraoperative use of inhalational anesthetics and narcotics.

3. Intraoperative anesthesia management

3.1 Monitoring

Standard monitoring recommended by the American Society of Anesthesiologists, such as two leads ECG, every 3 to 5 minutes measurement of noninvasive blood pressure and pulse oximetry is mandatory for intraoperative monitoring, especially if either LA or RA is primary anesthesia. If GA is an initial plan or required in the middle of the case for several reasons, close monitoring of BP (Blood Pressure) by invasive arterial line may be required due to cardiopulmonary comorbidities.

As to fluid administration, potassium-free crystalloids such as normal saline must be the first choice to reduce the possibility of intraoperative increases in potassium. It should be noted that potassium may increase so suddenly in the middle of the case even if preoperative potassium is at an acceptable level and/or the patient has a full HD one day before the surgery.

The surgery for HD access is not a major surgery and it barely loses blood. However, if the patient is anemic and vital signs become very unstable, especially in the case of GA, blood transfusion should be considered.

3.2 Potassium level

Any type of anesthesia may raise potassium to a critical level suddenly. Therefore, it is particularly important to pay close attention to ECG changes even for minor changes in the QRS complex or the height of the T wave. If recognized, the potassium level must be checked immediately. If elevated, immediate treatment to decrease the potassium should be initiated. Treatment for hyperkalemia starts with immediate administration of calcium (10 ml of 10% calcium chloride). A bolus dose of insulin (5–10 units while checking serum glucose simultaneously) should be followed by a continuous infusion of D10W with 5–10 units of regular insulin per 25–50 g of glucose. After this, sodium bicarbonate (50 to 100 mEq) and furosemide (if the patient still can make urine) should be administered. Other methods to decrease the potassium level includes increasing the respiration rate (if the patient's respiration is controllable under GA). Frequent checks of the potassium level should be performed until it is normalized.

3.3 Heparin

The surgeon will request heparin prior to clamping the artery. It is important to verify the dose of heparin by asking the surgeon again immediately before giving and flushing the lines to confirm the administration. We should inform the surgeon every hour after the initial and/or additional heparin is administered.

3.4 Oxygenation status

In cases undertaken with LA or RA where a patient is requiring high doses of sedatives, it can become difficult to maintain the patient of the airway. This can expose the patient to risk of hypoxia. In this situation, an adjunctive airway device can be placed with use of an oral or nasal airway or a conversion to GA with endotracheal tube or LMA should be considered to secure the airway. Since inserting an airway instrument, without muscle reluctance, is sometimes enough to stimulate the patient to move suddenly, the procedure should be paused during the intervention. It should be noted that the risk of bleeding during laryngoscopy and intubation is potentiated if the security of the airway is needed after heparin is administrated. Also, the possibility of potassium increase caused by respiratory acidosis during the patient's spontaneous respiration should be considered.

3.5 Choice of sedatives

A choice for sedatives during monitored anesthesia care is up to the anesthesiologist. However, we should consider the renal function of the patients is significantly impaired and that respiratory depression due to the sedatives may enhance to increase potassium due to respiratory acidosis. In addition to traditional sedatives, such as midazolam and fentanyl, relatively newer sedatives such as propofol, dexmedetomidine and remifentanil have been used to keep the patients calm and comfortable. The metabolism of propofol is not significantly affected by renal dysfunction and it remains a very popular one. However, it may cause respiratory depression if given at higher doses such as 100 micrograms/kg/min. If you need a higher dose, adding midazolam and/or fentanyl may be to reduce the dose. In terms of avoiding respiratory depression, dexmedetomidine is an excellent choice but may make systemic blood pressure lower than expected by decreasing HR. Even if lower BP may not happen during the surgery, it may happen in postoperative period due to a longer half-life of dexmedetomidine. A lower dose of remifentanil (less than 0.5 microgram/kg/min) can sedate the patients without inhibiting spontaneous respiration, but it may cause apnea if it is accidentally flushed. As described, any sedative has advantages and disadvantages of which the selection must be based on each individual patient's demand and background.

4. Postoperative anesthesia care

Anesthesia management does not discontinue at the end of the surgical procedure but when the patient is discharged from the postanesthesia care unit. It should be noted that potassium levels may increase suddenly even in the perioperative period. Therefore, the recovery nurse should pay close attention to ECG changes and possibly check the serum potassium if increase in potassium is suspected. Occasionally the timing of the next HD session may need to be advanced, especially for the patient that missed their regular HD session prior to the procedure. The criteria are varied between hospitals but consulting a nephrologist should be considered and common for any institute.

5. Updated topic: comparison of anesthesia type for patency, complications, and economy

Recently, the effect of anesthesia type on the patency of fistula, complications, and economy has been highlighted.

A previous retrospective study has reported that GA decreased early failure within 120 days after dialysis creation, while RA may decrease postoperative infection and bleeding [15]. On the other hand, a very recent study in 2022 did not show significant superiority of GA for fistula maturation [16].

The retrospective multivariable analysis has indicated that GA compared with RA/LA was independently associated with increased postoperative admission and decreased three months access utilization but similar 1-year access occlusion and intervention of which subgroup analysis of the RA/LA cohort showed RA was associated with increased three months access utilization but had similar 1-year access occlusion compared to LA [17]. A systematic review and meta-analysis comparison between RA and LA has indicated the superiority of RA over LA in terms of primary patency of fistula, brachial artery diameter, and operation duration [18]. A prospective study of the research group of Scotland, United Kingdom has indicated that RA significantly improved both primary and functional AVF patency at one year and cost compared to LA [19].

The topic of "which anesthesia is the best" has not been concluded yet. Most of the previous studies were retrospective or some were prospective but not enough of the subjects to conclude. Very recently, the new protocol of randomized, prospective, large-number study has been published [20]. The result of this study, which has not been opened yet as of November 2022, maybe promising and conclusive.

Author details

Koichiro Nandate
Harborview Medical Center, University of Washington, Seattle, WA, United States of America

*Address all correspondence to: knandate@uw.eduate

References

[1] Preoperative Tests. Clinical Guidelines. National institute for clinical excellence (NICE); 2003

[2] Wongyingsinn M, Suksuriyayothin S. Use of rapid ABG analyzer in measurement of potassium concentration: Does it agree with venous potassium concentration? Journal of the Medical Association of Thailand. 2009;**92**:925-929

[3] Kllerman PS. Preoperative care of the renal patient. Archives of Internal Medicine. 1994;**154**:1674-1688

[4] Brenowitz JB, Williams CD, Edwards WS. Major surgery in patients with chronic renal failure. Surgey. 1977;**134**:765-769

[5] Poli F, Scalamogna M, Cardillo M, Porta E, Sirchia G. An algorithm for cadaver kidney allocation based on a multivariate analysis of factors impacting on cadaver kidney graft survival and function. Transplant International. 2000;**13**:259-262

[6] Malinzak EB, Gan TJ. Regional anesthesia for vascular access surgery. Anesthesia and Analgesia. 2009;**109**:976-980

[7] Reynolds TS, Kim KM, Dukkipati R, Nguyen TH, Julka L, Kakazu C, et al. Pre-operative regional block anesthesia enhances operative strategy for arterilvenous fistula creation. The Journal of Vascular Access. 2010;**12**:336-340

[8] Shemesh D, Raikhinstein Y, Orkin D, Goldin I, Olsha O. Anesthesia for vascular access surgery. 2014;**15**:38-44

[9] Neal JM. Ultrasound-guided regional anesthesia and patient safety: An evidence-based analysis. Regional Anesthesia and Pain Medicine. 2010;**35**:59-67

[10] Sandhu N. Ultrasound imaging in anesthesia: An overview of vascular access and peripheral nerve blocks. Seminars in Anaesthesia Perioperative Medicine and Pain. 2007;**26**:197-209

[11] Sites BD, Brull R. Ultrasound guidance in peripheral regional anesthesia: Philosophy, evidence-based medicine and techniques. Current Opinion in Anaesthesiology. 2006;**19**:630-639

[12] Neal JM, Gerancher JC, Hebl JR, Iifeld BM, CJ MC, Franco CD, et al. Upper extremities regional anesthesia: Essentials of our current understanding, 2008. Regional Anesthesia and Pain Medicine. 2009;**34**:134-170

[13] Retzl G, Kapral S, Greher M, Mauritz W. Ultrasoongraphic findings of the axillary part of the brachial plexus. Anesth Anals. 2001;**92**:1271-1275

[14] Craig RG, Hunter JM. Recent developments in the perioperative management of adult patients with chronic kidney disease. British Journal of Anaesthesia. 2008;**101**:296-310

[15] Beaulieu RJ, Locham S, Nejim B, Dakour-Aridi H, Woo K, Malas MB. General anesthesia is associated with reduced early failure among patients undergoing hemodialysis access. Journal of Vascular Surgery. 2019;**69**:890-897

[16] Ramadan OI, Dember LM, Wang GJ, Ng JH, Mantell MP, Neuman MD. Association between anaesthesia type and arteriovenous fistula maturation. BMJ Open.

2022;**3**:100031. DOI: 10.1016/j.jjao.2022.100031

[17] Levin SR, Males MB, Tan TW, Conley CM, Salavati S, Arinze N, et al. Association of anesthesia type with outcomes after outpatient brachiocephalic arteriovenous fistula creation. Annals of Vascular Surgery. 2020;**68**:67-75

[18] Gao C, Weng C, He C, Xu J, Yu L. Comparison of reginal and local anesthesia for arteriovenous fistula creation in end-stage renal disease: A systematic review and meta-analysis. BMC Anesthesiology. 2020;**20**:219-226

[19] Aitken E, Kearns R, Gaianu L, Jackson A, Steven M, Kinsella J, et al. Long-term functional patency and cost effectiveness of arteriovenous fistula creation under regional anesthesia: A randomaized controlled trial. JASN. 2020;**31**:1871-1882

[20] Macfarlane A, Kearns RJ, Clancy MJ, Kingsmore D, Stevenson K, Jackson A, et al. The access collaborative group. Anaesthesia choice for creation of arteriovenous fistula (ACCess) study protocol: A randomized controlled trial comparing primary unassisted patency at one year of primary arteriovenous fistula creted under regional compared to local anaesthsia. BMJ Open. 2021;**11**:e052188. DOI: 10.1136/bmopen-2021-052188

Chapter 12

Artificial Liver Support Systems

Maiko Alejandro Tavera Díaz

Abstract

Acute liver failure and acute-on-chronic liver failure, regardless of the etiology, generate an inflammatory response in the liver parenchyma and systemic inflammatory response, as well as anti-inflammatory counterregulatory mechanisms that condition a state of immunomodulation, a condition that favors sepsis and septic shock. The increase in Von Willebrand factor and the increase in cellular traffic of monocytes and macrophages in the hepatic sinusoids, altering hepatic hemodynamics, is another mechanism of damage. Artificial liver support therapy represents an alternative in the support of these patients when medical treatment does not achieve the objectives. MARS, Prometheus, and SPAD favor detoxification. Plasma exchange and DPMAS are alternatives to limit the inflammatory response, eliminate Von Willebrand factor, and improve survival. Current evidence recommends the use of plasma exchange or combined extracorporeal support therapies as an alternative to achieve organ recovery or as a bridge to liver transplantation.

Keywords: acute liver failure, acute-on-chronic liver failure, artificial liver support systems, liver diseases, plasma exchange

1. Introduction

Liver diseases represent the tenth leading cause of death in the world and one of the leading causes of disability and years of life lost. Regardless of the etiology of liver disease, only 10% of those who require an organ get a transplant.

Acute liver failure and acute-on-chronic liver failure are serious pathologies, which despite the treatment of the cause and the associated complications, many of them require organ support through an artificial or biological system until the recovery of the liver is achieved. Liver support systems act as a bridge to liver transplantation [1].

2. Spectrum of liver diseases

Liver diseases are associated with poor outcomes and are often considered a medical emergency due to the severity and complications associated with mortality.

In the spectrum of the form of presentation, three entities are evident [2]:

1. Acute liver failure (ALF) in the context of health and normal liver function associated with a new noxa that determines the damage.

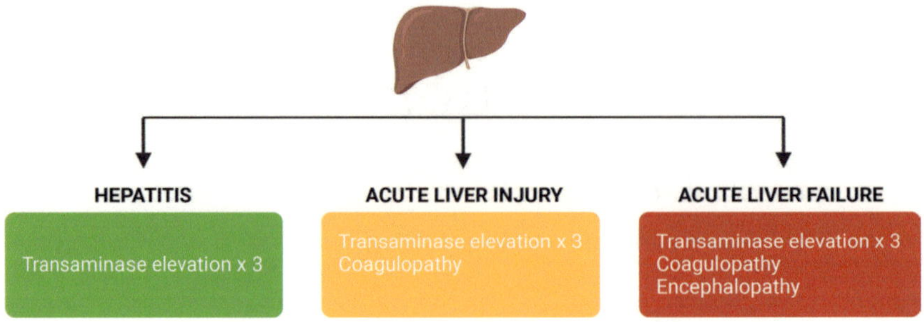

Figure 1.
Acute liver diseases are described: acute hepatitis, acute liver injury, and acute liver failure.

2. Acute-on-chronic liver failure (ACLF) develops on a background of chronic liver disease without cirrhosis or with underlying cirrhosis.

3. Known cirrhosis suffering from decompensation of liver function.

See **Figure 1**.

3. Acute liver failure

It represents a form of critical illness, potentially fatal, that occurs in 1 case per million, and the incidence is variable in each continent: Europe 0.62, Asia 6.2–23.8, USA 0.19 cases per 100,000 person-years [3]. The most frequent cause is paracetamol poisoning, followed by undetermined causes, drug-induced injury (DILI), and hepatitis [4].

Acute liver failure (ALF) represents severe liver damage (transaminase elevation x 3) with the development of hepatic encephalopathy preceded by jaundice. This time interval from jaundice to the presence of encephalopathy [5] allows its classification (**Table 1**):

Author	O'grady	AIEH
Hyperacute	1–7 days	< 10 days
Acute	8–28 days	10–30 days
Subacute	5–12 weeks	5–24 weeks
Chronic	> 26 weeks	> 24 weeks

Table 1.
Classifications of acute liver failure, which correspond to the time interval from the onset of jaundice to the development of encephalopathy.

4. Acute on chronic liver failure

The development of acute liver failure on chronic failure (ACLF) occurs at any stage of the spectrum of chronic liver disease without cirrhosis or with compensated or decompensated liver cirrhosis [6], in which there are one or several precipitating

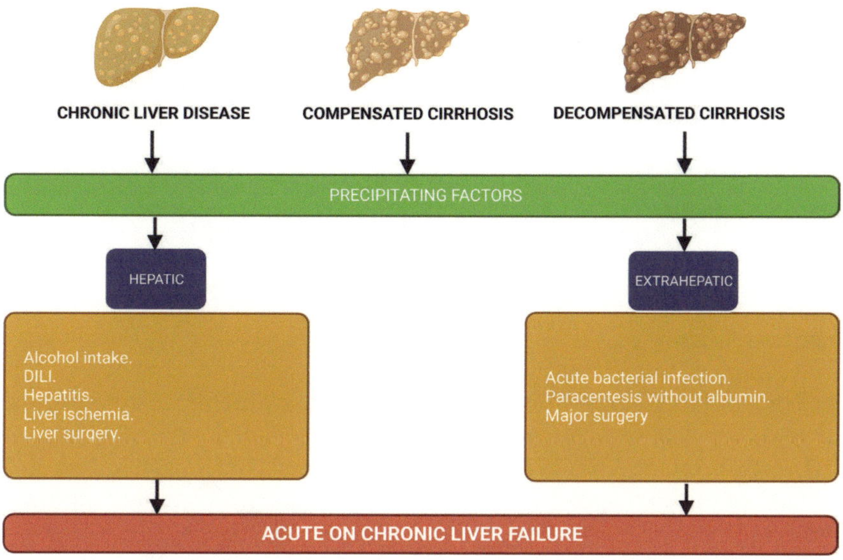

Figure 2.
In the spectrum of chronic liver disease without cirrhosis or with compensated or decompensated liver cirrhosis, the clinical condition that favors exposure to a hepatic or extrahepatic precipitant generates an inflammatory response that induces the development of multiple organ failure.

events in the liver (alcohol ingestion, DILI, hepatitis, hepatic ischemia, liver surgery) or extrahepatic (acute bacterial infection, paracentesis without albumin, major surgery), which cause the development of multiple organ failure with the increased mortality between 28 and 90 days (**Figure 2**) [7].

There is no universal definition, there are at least four consensuses that define it and the prevalence differs from continent to continent, in USA 10, EU 20.1, ASIA 5.1 cases per 1000 person-years [8].

The most agreed definitions of ACLF are mentioned below: (**Table 2**) [7],

The severity of ACLF is measured by the degree of organic dysfunction through the CLIF-SOFA score in different cohorts of three subjects (CANONIC, PREDICT, KACLIF, COSSH, MAHMUD, HERNAEZ) showing us that the analytical alteration

APASL	EASL-CLIF	NACSELD	WGO
Acute liver damage manifesting as Jaundice (BT 5 mg/dl) and coagulopathy (INR > 1.5), complicated within 4 weeks with ascites and encephalopathy in a patient with diagnosed or undiagnosed chronic liver disease.	Pre-existing CLD acute deterioration, related to a precipitating event associated with multiorgan failure with high mortality at 28 and 90 days.	Syndrome characterized by acute deterioration in a patient with cirrhosis, due to an infection, developing failure of two or more extrahepatic organs.	Syndrome in CLD with or without previously diagnosed cirrhosis is characterized by acute hepatic decompensation, resulting in liver failure (jaundice and prolonged INR) and failure of one or more extrahepatic organs with high mortality at 28 and 90 days.

Asian Pacific Association for the Study of the Liver (APASL), European Association for the Study of Chronic Liver Failure (EASL-Clif), North American Consortium for the Study of End-Stage Liver Disease's definition of acute-on-chronic liver failure, and World Gastroenterology Organization (WGO).

Table 2.
Characteristics of definitions of ACLF developed by four different consortia.

is significant insofar as to the presence of leukocytosis, PCR, increases in TNF alpha, and IL-8 in statistically significant values in patients with ACLF when compared with decompensated or compensated cirrhosis. Likewise, it is observed that transplant-free mortality is higher in patients with ACLF [8].

5. Pathophysiology

5.1 Inflammatory response

5.1.1 Acute liver failure

Regardless of the etiology of liver damage, apoptosis and hepatocyte necrosis are generated, which allows the release of damage-associated molecular patterns (DAMPs), such as micro-RNA 122, high mobility protein 1 (HMGB1), Keratin 18, which bind to toll-like receptors (TLR4) of Kupffer cells, which induces the release of cytokines.

Activation of the Kupffer cells induces the release of cytokines, which stimulates the recruitment of monocytes and induces an intrahepatic inflammatory phenotype, with sequestration of platelets and amplifying the inflammatory response. The inflammatory process is not limited to the liver, this induces a systemic inflammatory response (SIRS), and a counterregulatory mechanism called compensatory anti-inflammatory response syndrome (CARS) is induced, the latter conditions a state of immunomodulation, which explains the high risk of infections, risk of sepsis, multi-organ failure, and worsening of encephalopathy (**Figure 3**) [9].

Neopterin formed by macrophages, monocytes, and activated dendritic cells has been described; it is considered a marker of inflammation in ALF due to

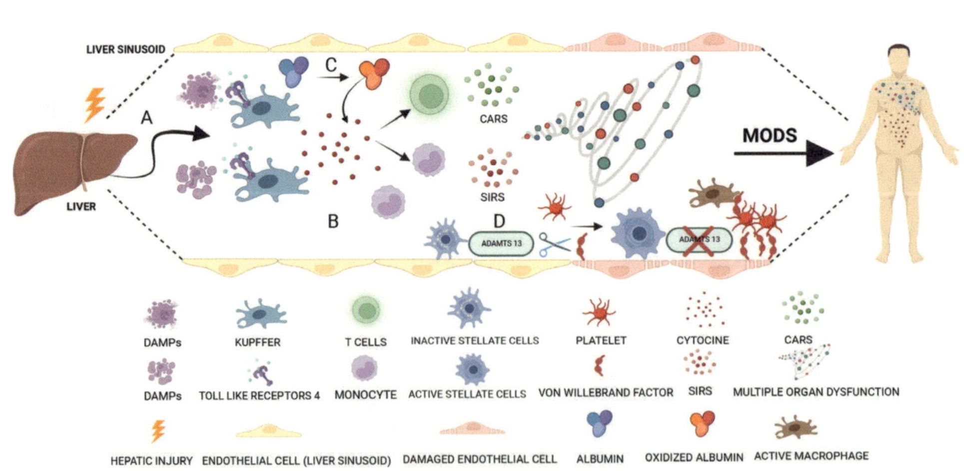

Figure 3.
A) Regardless of the etiology of the liver injury, the release of DAMPs is generated, recognized by the TLR4 of Kupffer cells. B) Activated Kupffer cells release cytokines, which stimulate monocyte migration, amplifying the inflammatory response within the liver. C) Inflammation is not limited to this organ and generates SIRS; likewise, a counterregulatory mechanism (CARS) is stimulated, which leads to a state of immunoparalysis and increases the risk of infections. D) Albumin in its oxidized form contributes to the perpetuation of the inflammatory state. E) Damage to the stellate cells of the hepatic sinusoids decreases the release of ADAMTS 13, increases the expression of VWF multimers, favors platelet aggregation that predisposes to the formation of microthrombi, and, together with the increase in monocyte and macrophage trafficking, alters hepatic circulation.

acetaminophen. It is evident that the increase in neopterin and sCD163 correlates with SIRS, greater clinical severity measured by SOFA score, and with the requirement of liver transplantation [10]. The aforementioned supports the increase in mononuclear cell activity and the increase in the inflammatory response in ALF.

Acute liver failure has great potential to develop multi-organ complications (cerebral, respiratory, metabolic, hematological, hemodynamic, infectious, and renal) despite supportive management, many of them do not stabilize and lead to an increase in mortality. In this critical condition, extracorporeal liver support therapies are used until the recovery of liver function, which, in some series, reaches 60% of acute patients and without reaching transplantation [11].

5.1.2 Acute chronic liver failure

It represents the spectrum of chronic liver disease without cirrhosis or with compensated or decompensated cirrhosis, in which a hepatic or extrahepatic precipitating factor triggers a persistent inflammatory response that induces the development.

TNF alpha and activated stellate cells, allowing nitric oxide secretion, further damage hepatocytes and cause splanchnic vasodilation. The endothelin released from endothelial cells decreases the expression of cluster of differentiation (CD) and human leukocyte anti-DR (HLA), conditions an environment of TL reg inhibition, and lowers LTH 17 activation. This conditions a state of "Ineffective Immunity," dysfunctional cells, decreased phagocytic activity, increased anti-inflammatory cytokines, and release of reactive oxygen species (ROS) [12].

ACLF conditions a SIRS state in the first 7 days from the onset of the symptoms and after 10–14 days, a state of immunosuppression due to anti-inflammatory

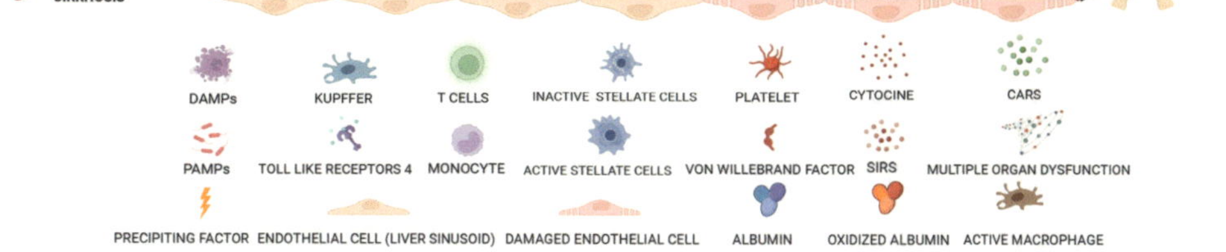

Figure 4.
A) In chronic liver disease without cirrhosis and in compensated or decompensated cirrhosis, they generate the favorable environment for the arrival of PAMPs in the enterohepatic circulation, mitochondrial stress, apoptosis, and necrosis typical of liver disease, regardless of the etiology, allowing the release of DAMPs. Both molecules bind to TRL4 receptors of Kupffer cells, which are activated and release cytokines with hepatic and systemic impact. B) The intrahepatic inflammatory response and the release of chemokines induce chemotaxis of monocyte-derived macrophages from the systemic circulation to the liver at sites of injury. C) Albumin in the oxidized form contributes to the perpetuation of the inflammatory state. D) Damage to the stellate cells of the hepatic sinusoids decreases the release of ADAMTS 13 and increases the expression of VWF multimers that favors platelet aggregation and stimulates phagocytosis of these molecules by macrophages, increasing cell size and increasing the number of cells. Cell traffic contributes to lower liver perfusion.

cytokines (CARS) is generated, increasing the risk of sepsis, septic shock, and multiple organ failure (**Figure 4**) [13].

The severity of ACLF measured by CLIF-SOFA has a direct relationship with mortality. The measures used in the management with crystalloid solutions and human albumin, and the use of vasoactive agents are a necessity to meet the hemodynamic objectives, anti-encephalopathy measures, and anti-cerebral edema. The need for transfusion of blood products and the support of mechanical ventilation and infection control represent the supportive management of these patients. Many of them, despite the optimization of the measures implemented, require extracorporeal liver support therapy, which, as in acute liver failure, has the clear objective of limiting the inflammatory response that perpetuates cell damage, decreasing macrophage activation that conditions the permanent inflammatory response.

5.2 Oxidation of albumin

Albumin is a high molecular weight protein (MW 66.5 kD), which is a fundamental determinant since it provides 75% of the oncotic pressure, necessary to maintain fluids in the intravascular compartment, and represents 54% of the plasma proteins, with a hepatic synthesis rate of 150 m/kg/day [14]. Albumin is formed by a polypeptide chain of 585 amino acids, divided into three domains I, II and III. Each domain is subdivided in types A and B, it is composed of 35 cysteine residues, of which 34 residues form 17 disulfide bridges and leave the cysteine residue (Cys) 34 free to interact with others molecules (**Table 3**) [15].

The important functions of albumin include being a regulator of extracellular fluids, it allows the reversible transport of endogenous products, such as fat-soluble hormones and free fatty acids, transporting unconjugated bilirubin, and exogenous products such as metals, drugs, and drugs. It also fulfills a function important in PH control, buffering non-volatile acids, and competitive binding to calcium ions. Antioxidant properties are described because it is a source of reduced sulfhydryl groups with properties to eliminate ROS, with anti-inflammatory and endothelial protection effects [14].

Albumin mostly circulates in a reduced state, called human mercaptoalbumin (HMA) with a free thiol group at residue Cys 34, to which ROS and nitrogen bind, allowing their uptake and removal of free radicals. Albumin can undergo several post-translational modifications in physiological or pathological conditions, which undergoes oxidation through disulfide bonding between Cys34 and sulfhydryl-containing compounds such as glutathione, homocysteine, and cysteine. This reversibly oxidized form of albumin is called non-mercaptoalbumin type 1 (HNA-1) and the complete and irreversible oxidation of Cys 34 albumin to sulfonic or sulfinic acid confers the

Domain I	Domain II	Domain III	CYS 34
Uremic toxins Thyroxin Warfarin	Halotan Propofol Ibuprofen Uremic toxins Thyroxin	Bilirubin Hemin Doxorubicin	Nitric oxide

Table 3.
Each albumin domain allows the transport of different substances, and the CYS 34 residue has the capacity to eliminate ROS.

name non-mercaptoalbumin type 2 (HNA-2) [16, 17]. Other forms of modified albumin are also described, such as ischemia-modified albumin (IMA), in which it undergoes a conformational change in the N-terminal portion, decreasing the metal transport capacity, and the IMA/albumin ratio is also increased in patients. with cirrhosis and ACLF, described as a marker associated with higher mortality. Other forms of cystei-nylated, glycated and truncated modified alumina are mentioned, all the described forms of oxidized albumin lose the capacity to transport molecules and detoxify, increasing the free component of many toxic substances that alter the functions of organs and systems [17].

The expression of non-mercaptoalbumin types 1 and 2 has an effect on the activation of mononuclear cells by stimulating the release of cytokines (IL 1β, IL 6, IL 8, and TNF-α), amplifying or perpetuating the inflammatory response, by which a relationship between the levels of oxidized albumin and the pro-inflammatory state exists. In a cohort study of 79 patients, non-mercaptoalbumin type 1 phosphorylated the mitogen-activated protein kinase (MAP) p38α [18] was observed, which increases the activity of the transcription factor NF-κB, induces the production of cytokines, and also increases the production of inflammatory COX2 eicosanoides such as thromboxane A 2 (TXA2), leukotriene B 4 (LTB4), and prostaglandin G2 (PG2) [18].

We see that albumin oxidation is a mechanism that by itself induces and perpetuates inflammation in patients with decompensated cirrhosis and acute-on-chronic liver failure, which opens the way for the search for other applications of extracorporeal liver support therapies.

In a randomized crossover design trial of eight patients with ACLF, who underwent alternate eight treatments with MARS and Prometheus, non-mercaptoalbumin types 1 and 2 levels were measured and found to be elevated, and there was a transient change in status redox, from non-mercaptoalbumin to mercaptoalbumin that lasted a short time, returning to the oxidized forms of albumin after 24 hours [19].

There are few studies that evaluate extracorporeal liver support techniques as an alternative for albumin detoxification or regeneration. The Molecular Adsorbent Recirculating System (MARS) was found to be useful in removing substances bound to albumin and improving hepatic encephalopathy, but in a small study of 34 MARS patients [20], it did not show benefit in improving functional capacity or regenerating capacity and normal functionality of albumin. It is possible that liver damage and inflammation lead to irreversible damage to albumin and extracorporeal liver support techniques based only on albumin recirculation with small-capacity and easily saturated adsorbents.

5.3 Von Willebrand factor and ADAMTS 13 effect on ALF and ACLF

The Von Willebrand factor (VWF) is formed by endothelial cells, megakaryocytes, and hepatocytes in the latter when the hepatic injury occurs [21]. This factor is cleared by macrophages and stored in endothelial cells, in Weibel-Palade bodies, and in the alpha granules of megariocytes.

VWF has MW 10,000 KD and is released at sites of vascular damage in response to secretion stimuli, such as thrombin, endothelial stress, vasopressin, or its synthetic analog desmopressin.

In ALF and ACLF, it generates damage to the endothelial cells of the liver sinusoids and releases VWF multimers, which bind to Domain A1, Glycoprotein IB Alpha (GPIbα), and GPIIb/IIa of platelets, and subendothelial collagen, allowing adhesion, platelet aggregation, and sequestration, giving rise to the formation of microthrombi and generating intrahepatic hemodynamic changes and liver ischemia, cell necrosis, worsening of liver function, activating innate immunity, and contributing to the development of multi-organ dysfunction [22].

Basic experimentation studies in mice with ALF by paracetamol show an increase in VWF and platelet aggregation after 48 hours after drug exposure [21, 23]. In a prospective study of patients with ACLF, increased VWF was correlated with higher MELD and SOFA scores [22].

Damage to stellate cells determines a lower release of ADAMTS 13. Under normal conditions, this disintegrin metalloproteinase cleaves the TYr 1605-Met 1606 bond of the VWF A2 domain, degrading the VWF multimers. In ALF and ACLF, low levels of ADAMTS 13 [24, 25] are identified, causing less cleavage of the VWF multimeters. These new links require further studies on the use of VWF inhibitors, ADAMTS 13 supplementation, or the use of extracorporeal liver support therapies for the removal of VWF multimers [25] and limiting liver damage.

5.4 Macrophage activation

When hepatocyte damage is generated, Kupffer cells express two phenotypes: proinflammatory where Kupffer cells release cytokines (IL-1β, tumor necrosis factor (TNF)-α and Ccl2), the chemokine Ccl2 and the activity of plasmin during liver tissue damage, stimulating the chemotaxis of monocyte-derived macrophages from the systemic circulation to the liver at sites of injury, in order to control intrahepatic trafficking, endocytosis, phagocytosis, and phenotype switching to one of repair with dedifferentiation of macrophages to fibroblasts [26].

Under healthy conditions, macrophages constitutively present CD163 and CD206 receptors. During the proinflammatory phase of ALF and ACLF, a detachment of soluble sCD163 and sCD206 is generated, and the severity of ALF, ACLF, and mortality is considered biomarkers [27], which may play a role in making early medical or transplant decisions.

Macrophages are persistently activated in the presence of VWF and these cells are located in low-pressure sinusoids, being the parking residence of activated macrophages and which, together with microthrombi, alter hepatic hemodynamics.

The lines of study in inhibitors of macrophage chemotaxis, the use of extracorporeal liver purification therapies in the elimination of cytokines and chemokines, and achieving immunomodulation that allows limiting the migration of mononuclear cells to the liver and mitigates the damage may be promising.

5.5 Extracorporeal liver support therapy

Liver support therapies have been used with the aim of trying to replace the loss of important functions of the liver, and these systems are limited to detoxification and to reduce the inflammatory response.

5.5.1 Types of extracorporeal liver support therapy

They are divided into artificial and biological [28]. In this review, the description of artificial therapies will be made (**Table 4**).

The artificial liver support system allows the removal of water-soluble toxins, such as ammonium, urea, creatinine, iron, aromatic amino acids, trypophan, and also fat-soluble toxins, such as bile acids, conjugated and unconjugated bilirubin, short and

Artificial	Biological
1. MARS 2. Fractionated plasma separation and adsorption (Prometheus) 3. Single-pass albumin dialysis (SPAD). 4. Hemoperfusion 5. Plasma exchange 6. Plasma adsorption 7. Double plasma molecular absorption system (DPMAS)	1. ELAD® 2. BiologicDT 3. Hepa-Mate™ 4. TEAK-BALSS/HBAL 5. AMC-BAL 6. HEPATASSIST SYSTEM

Table 4.
Classification of liver support systems.

medium chain fatty acids, benzoadiazepines endogenous, mercaptans, copper, nitric oxide, indoyxisulfate, and protoporphyrin [29].

We consider that the removal of the mentioned toxicants with detoxification-only approach does not generate the clear benefit due to the extensive mechanisms of perpetuation of liver damage, it is possible that the traditional MARS, Prometheus techniques are not good enough due to the smaller diameter of the beads, smaller pore diameter, smaller amount of resin, and smaller adsorbent surface in the first two and that the concentration of albumin used in MARS and SPAD is not sufficient, and these details will be reviewed in each of the techniques extracorporeal support.

5.5.2 When to start extracorporeal liver support therapy?

The most agreed recommendations for the start of extracorporeal support are the following [30]:

1. Severe acute liver injury regardless of cause.

2. Acute liver failure regardless of cause.

3. Acute on chronic liver failure.

4. Sepsis with severe liver injury.

5. Acute kidney injury with criteria for hepatorenal syndrome that does not respond to treatment with Terlipressin and albumin.

6. Primary nonfunction and delayed graft function following liver transplantation.

7. Delayed graft function in simultaneous liver kidney transplantation.

8. Post-hepatectomy liver failure.

9. Hypoxic liver injury.

10. Refractory pruritus.

5.5.3 Artificial extracorporeal liver support systems

5.5.3.1 Molecular adsorbent recirculating system (MARS)

This purification system allows the elimination of toxins bound to albumin and water-soluble toxins. The blood that is extracted by catheter circulates at a blood flow of 200 ml/min and is placed in contact with the high permeability MARS® FLUX 2.1 filter (60 kD) and 600 ml of dialysate albumin circulates counter currently with pumped 150 ml/min. This recirculated albumin is placed in contact with the diaFLUX 1.8 filter and with the conventional dialysis bath of the Prismaflex System, allowing the elimination of water-soluble molecules, and the regenerated albumin circulates through the activated carbon cartridge (diaMARS® AC250) that captures cationic toxins and then goes to a second resin cartridge (diaMARS® IE250) that captures anionic toxins. The procedure is performed with an average of 8 hours up to date, with the aim of reducing total bilirubin by more than 25% in each session, achieving a reduction in nitrogen and ammonia and reversing encephalopathy (**Figure 5**).

In the FULMAR study [31], a randomized control trial (RCT), a multicenter study that included 102 ALFs on the liver transplant waiting list, of which standard medical treatment (SMT) vs. SMT and MARS were compared, in this study, it was seen that overall survival at 6 months, transplant-free survival at 6 months, and survival at 1 year were not significantly different in both groups, but transplant-free survival was better in those patients who received more than 3 MARS sessions ($p = 0.001$) when compared to STM. In relation to other outcomes, there was no improvement in encephalopathy between both treatment groups, but a significant decrease in bilirubin, creatinine, and lactate values was achieved compared to SMT, and it is a valuable therapy in patients who are not candidates for liver transplantation.

In the RELIEF study [32], a multicenter RCT, recruited 189 patients with decompensated cirrhosis (total bilirubin > 5 mg/dl, hepatorenal syndrome or hepatic encephalopathy grade II) and compared STM vs MARS and STM treatment, there

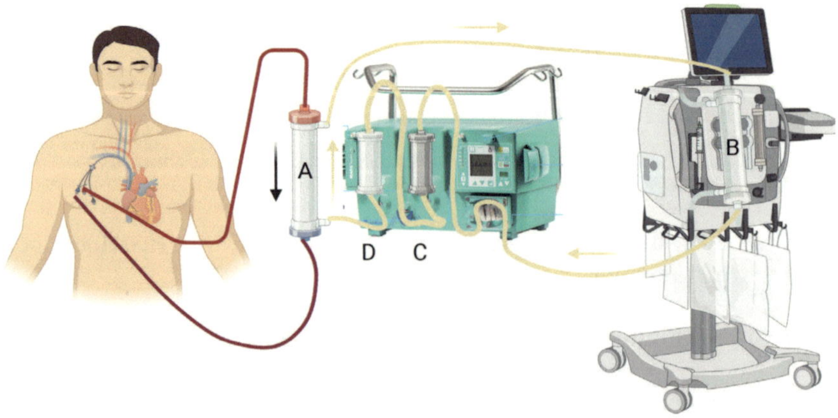

Figure 5.
Molecular adsorbent recirculating system (MARS). A) Once the patient's blood enters the high permeability (60 kD) MARS® FLUX 2.1 filter, 600 ml of dialysate albumin circulates in a countercurrent direction with pumped 150 ml/min. B) Then, the recirculated albumin is directed to the diaFLUX 1.8 filter and with the conventional dialysis bath of the Prismaflex system, allowing the elimination of water-soluble molecules. C) Next, the regenerated albumin circulates through the activated carbon cartridge (diaMARS® AC250) that captures cationic toxins. D) It is then directed to a second resin cartridge (diaMARS® IE250).

were no differences in survival at 28 and 90 days, in the survival analysis by subgroups there were no differences in survival either, without differences in the length of stay in intensive care and hospital stay, but a significant decrease in bilirubin and creatinine values was achieved in favor of therapy MARS. The lack of evidence is attributed, whether it is related to the heterogeneity in the definition of ACLF, small sample size, low dose of therapy, rapid saturation of the cartridges and albumin, or that MARS therapy does not adjust to the severity of many patients.

A meta-analysis published by Arjun Vaid et al. [33] review 10 RCT and one no RCT and use the Jadad scale to assess the quality of the studies, recruited patients, including ALF and ACLF, and receive MARS from one to 10 sessions, lasting between 6 and 8 hours. The outcomes show a significant decrease in bilirubin levels ($p = < 0.001$), there was also improvement in encephalopathy ($p = <0.001$), but MARS therapy did not reduce mortality ($p = 0.62$), in the analysis by subgroups when performing more than three sessions or increasing the concentration of albumin >20%, which did not influence the reduction of mortality.

Rafael Banares et al. [34], published a high-intensity MARS meta-analysis, recruited 285 patients with ACLF and called high-intensity MARS when they received more than 5 sessions. In the high intensity group, 10-day survival ($p = 0.001$) and 30 days ($p = 0.041$) is higher and there was a significant decrease in the MELD score, bilirubin, creatinine, and encephalopathy improvement, compared to the low intensity group, when the number of sessions was less than 5 MARS sessions.

One recently published DELPHI consensus of international experts [35] recommends extracorporeal albumin dialysis (ECAD) in the MARS modality should be started in the early stages of grade II encephalopathy or within 24–48 hours of refractory hepatic encephalopathy and when indications for liver transplantation are present and more than 3 sessions lasting 8 hours are recommended. The reported evidence mention improvement in survival at 21 days in ACL due to acetaminophen, but no benefit at 6–12 months. The use of ECAD is not recommended in patients in the late stages of ALF where multiple organ dysfunction is already expressed.

6. Prometheus

It is a fractionated plasma separation and adsorption system, the blood extracted through a catheter circulates through an AlbuFlow® AF01 filter, with a high screening coefficient (250 kD), which separates the albumin from the blood, the first to pass through the plasma to an adsorbent cartridge Prometh® 01 contains a neutrally charged, highly porous resin that absorbs bile acids, aromatic amino acids, and phenols. Then, the plasma and the albumin circulate through a second Prometh® 02 cartridge, which is an anion exchange resin in the form of chloride that allows the absorption of bilirubin, and following the sequence of the circuit, the blood plasma and the detoxified albumin are returned to the Fresenius® helixone high-flow filter to remove water-soluble toxins (**Figure 6**).

In the HELIOS study [36], an RCT included 145 patients with ACLF and compared SMT vs. SMT and Prometheus, in the survival outcomes at 28–90 days there were no statistical differences, the mean until death had no differences, and the severity of MELD and encephalopathy improved in the Prometheus group, in the univariate analysis there was no improvement in survival in patients with hepatorenal syndrome, the length of stay in critical care and the hospital was similar in both groups, and in the analytical the only value that improved it was the bilirubin.

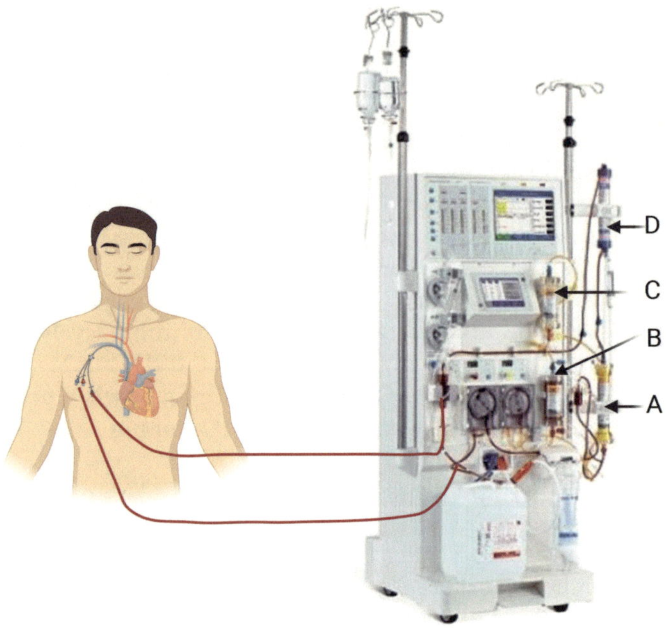

Figure 6.
Fractionated plasma separation and adsorption (Prometheus). A) The blood extracted through a catheter circulates through an AlbuFlow ® AF01 filter. B) Albumin and separated plasma pass to a Prometh® 01 adsorbent cartridge. C) Albumin then circulates through a second Prometh® 02 cartridge. D) Following the circuit sequence, blood plasma and detoxified albumin are returned to the Fresenius® helixone high-flow filter.

7. Mars and prometheus theory combination

In a randomized crossover design study, eight patients with ACLF who underwent MARS and Prometheus on alternate days were evaluated, completing 17 sessions for each of the two artificial liver support systems. Cytokine measurements were performed in healthy controls and in patients with ACLF, evidencing elevated IL-6, IL-8, IL-10, TNF-α, and sTNF-αR1 values in the latter group. This work shows that there was no significant decrease in cytokines at the end of treatment and other reviews with both artificial support systems report similar results. The low efficiency is attributed to the high rate of cytokine production due to multiple mechanisms of the perpetuation of the inflammatory response, the greater saturation of the cartridges, or less adsorbent capacity [37–39].

8. Single-pass albumin dialysis (SPAD)

This purification system that uses the physical foundation of diffusion with a dialysis bath enriched with albumin in 3–4% concentrations that act as a binder for substances bound to proteins. This technique uses a continuous renal replacement therapy (CRRT) machine in continuous venovenous hemodialysis modality, with a dialysate flow of 700–1000 ml/min. The dialysate flow with albumin will allow the capture of lipophilic molecules present in the patient's blood that will bind to the albumin that circulates in the countercurrent direction to the blood flow through the filter, allowing the elimination of bilirubin, bile acids, and nitrogen acids (**Figure 7**).

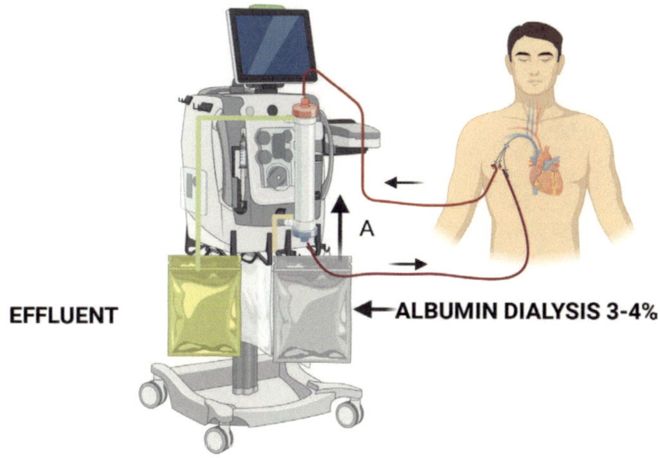

Figure 7.
Single-pass albumin dialysis (SPAD). A) The technique uses a continuous renal replacement therapy (CRRT) machine in continuous venovenous hemodialysis modality, with a dialysate flow of 700–1000 ml/min, the dialysate is enriched with 3–4% albumin.

This technique does not use additional cartridges or other extracorporeal circulation machines and can be performed in low-income countries.

There is evidence that SPAD allows a significant decrease in bilirubin similar to MARS, but it failed to lower bile acid and cytokine values [40], considering that the modality used is continuous venovenous hemodialysis and due to the screening coefficient of conventional membranes does not allow clearance of cytokines [41].

In a randomized crossover trial [42], of 34 patients with ACLF, who underwent dialysis with albumin, assigning the first session randomly to MARS or SPAD modality, the second session was assigned to a different therapy. Both therapies achieve a significant decrease in bilirubin, bile acids, and a greater decrease in creatinine with MARS. The significant decrease in fibrinogen in SPAD was identified as an adverse effect, and both therapies decreased hemoglobin, hematocrit, and platelets. Both therapies are considered comparable, with the advantage of the lower costs of SPAD.

9. Plasma exchange

The plasma exchange (PE) is an extracorporeal purification technique that is carried out by centrifugation or filtration. This last technique uses a high permeability membrane with a large pore size greater than 0.3 microns, allowing the separation of plasma and the removal of medium and medium molecules with high molecular weight, such as cytokines and immunoglobulins (**Figure 8**).

Within the pathophysiological mechanisms of acute and chronic liver injury, the increase in Von Willebrand multimeters stands out due to a decrease in the release of ADAMTS 13 as a result of stellate cell damage. The increase in the Von Willebrand factor multimeters intervenes in platelet aggregation in the hepatic sinusoids and conditions the migration of macrophages for their phagocytosis, and both alterations condition a deterioration of the vascular flow of the liver and also condition a greater inflammatory response.

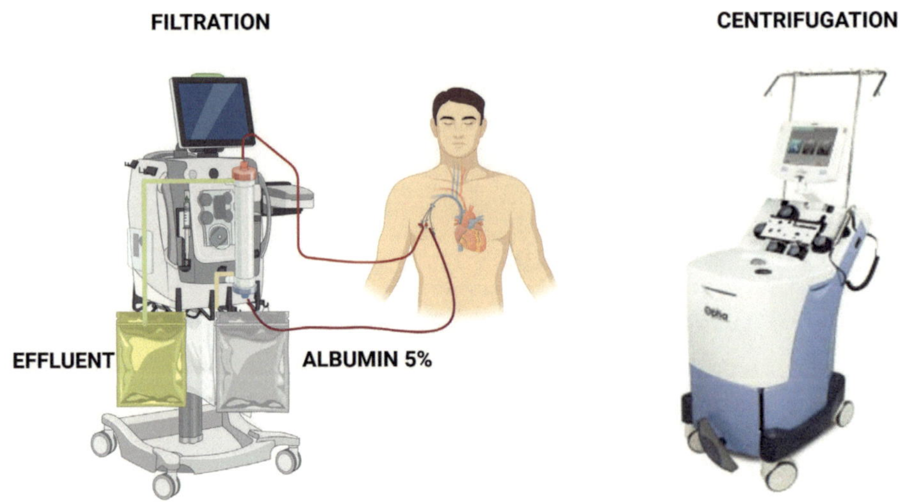

Figure 8.
Plasma exchange (PE). The technique uses a high permeability membrane with a large pore size that allows plasma separation and replacement of the extracted volume is performed with 5% albumin or fresh frozen plasma.

Klaus Stahl et al. [43], in a single-center prospective study, demonstrated in 31 patients with sepsis that plasma exchange increased ADAMTS 13 activity and decreased VWF antigen, confirming the therapeutic application of this imbalance.

The RCT described by Larsen et al. [44], through an RCT in 182 patients with ALF, evaluated SMT vs. SMT and high volume plasma exchange for 3 days (8–12 L) with replacement with fresh-frozen plasma in equivalent volume. In the consulted evidence, the primary outcome that corresponds to liver transplant-free survival during the hospital stay was higher in the group that received plasma exchange (p = 0.0083), and survival in those who did not receive a transplant and received plasma exchange was better when compared with those who were not transplanted and did not receive plasma exchange. In the group with plasma exchange, the hemodynamic variables improved, noradrenaline doses were reduced, the SOFA and Clif SOFA severity scores improved, and the analysis showed improvement in coagulation times, decreased bilirubin, alanine aminotransferase (ALT), and ammonium. When the inflammatory response is assessed, plasma exchange reduces DAMPs, TNF alpha, IL 16 at 48 hours, and IL 18, and decreases in CD 163, CD 64, and CCR7, which indicates less mononuclear cell traffic.

High-volume plasma exchange carries risks with high replacement volume and could worsen cerebral edema, Maiwall et al. [45], report a prospective open-label RCT study where 40 patients with ALF were recruited, each group was divided into 20 patients for SMT vs STM and standard plasma exchange (1–1.5 plasma volumes per PE session). The outcome of transplant-free survival at 21 days was higher in the group with plasma exchange (p 0.04). In the secondary outcomes, there is evidence of a lower inflammatory response and a smaller diameter of the optic nerve sheath with a predictor of decreased cerebral edema, hemodynamic variables, vascular resistance index improved, SOFA score decreased, there was a decrease in lactate and bilirubin values they also decreased. When inflammation data are analyzed, a decrease in innate immunity cytokines and an increase in anti-inflammatory cytokines, a significant decrease in DAMPs, endotoxins, and a decrease in VWF are evident in the group that received exchange plasma.

In a retrospective study [46] of 50 patients with alcohol-related acute on chronic liver failure (A-ACLF), low-dose corticosteroid treatment was compared

Points	Liver cirrhosis	Total bilirubin (μmol/L)	PT-INR	Infection	Hepatic encephalopathy
0	No	< 425	< 2.0	Non-spontaneous bacterial peritonitis (SBP)	No
1	And it is	425–650	2.0–2.5	Yes SBP	I–II
2	And it is	≥ 650	≥ 2.5	SBP plus other site infection	III–IV

Table 5.
PALS score predictive score of short-term prognosis for patients treated with plasma exchange.

with low-volume plasma exchange (LVPE) (0.5–1 plasma volumes per PE session) vs. SMT, Kaplan-Meier survival analysis shows better survival in the first year (P = 0.03) and there were lower levels of VWF in the plasma exchange group. Further large randomized control trials are needed to evaluate the efficacy of LVPE in ACLF.

In a systematic review and meta-analysis [47] of 16 RCTs that included 1670 patients with ALF, the efficiency of each therapy was compared to SMT, ELAD, MARS, Prometheus, and plasma exchange. It is shown that the probability of having greater overall survival at the first and third month as well as transplant-free survival at 3 months was better with exchange plasma.

The European Association for the Study of the Liver [11], in the guidelines for the management of acute liver failure, recommends plasma exchange improves transplant-free survival and modulates immune dysfunction with evidence level I, grade of recommendation 1. and recommends early onset and in those who will not undergo liver transplantation with evidence level I, grade of recommendation 2.

One DELPHI consensus of international experts [35] recently published, in relation to PEHV, is recommended due to the greater transplant-free and in-hospital survival. The PLAS score [48] uses two derivation and validation cohorts of patients with ACLF, whose predictive value for 3-month mortality when the score was greater than 6 points (AUC 0.80 derivation cohort and 0.78 validation cohort) has better performance when it is compared with the model for end-stage liver disease (MELD) and also with other mortality scores. The variables taken into account for stratification are liver cirrhosis total bilirubin, PT-INR, infection, and hepatic encephalopathy. The score goes from a minimum of 0 to a maximum of 9, it is called grade I: score of 0–2, grade II: 3–5, grade III: 6–9 (**Table 5**).

Extracorporeal liver support therapy is not recommended in patients who develop platelet counts <40,000/mm3, INR > 2.5, and fibrinogen <1 g/L, which would increase the risk of bleeding [35].

10. Plasma adsorption perfusion

Plasma adsorption perfusion (PAP) uses a CRRT or intermittent hemodialysis machine. Once the blood comes out through the catheter with a blood pump flow at 150 ml/min, it allows the blood to enter the plasma exchange filter where it allows the separation of the plasma by filtration. The obtained plasma is mobilized by a second

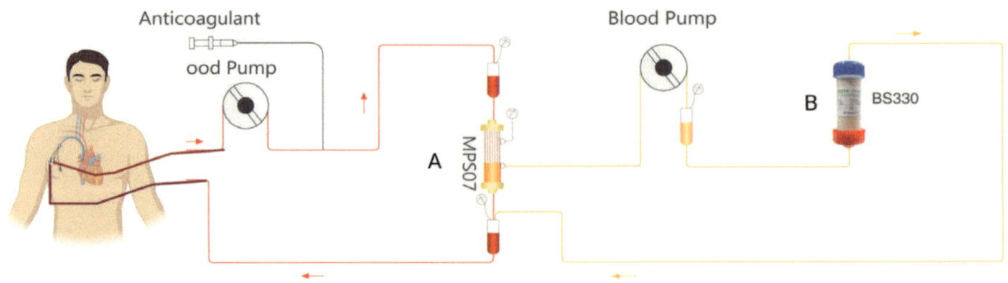

Figure 9.
Plasma adsorption perfusion (PAP). A) The blood exits through the catheter with a blood pump flow at 150 ml/min, it allows the blood to enter the plasma exchange filter where it allows the separation of the plasma by filtration. B) The obtained plasma is mobilized by a second pump at 25–50 ml/min and enters a cartridge made of the styrene-divinylbenzene copolymer.

pump at 25–50 ml/min and enters a cartridge made of styrene-divinylbenzene copolymer, with the capacity to adsorb bilirubin, bile acids, and cytokines. This technique has some advantages over the other techniques mentioned, such as it does not require the use of exogenous plasma or albumin infusion, it does not eliminate coagulation factors, and it is less expensive than MARS (**Figure 9**).

A single-center retrospective study [49] evaluated the performance of three therapies (MARS, PAP, and PE) and recruited 103 patients with hyperbilirubinemia due to ALF and ACLF, and extracorporeal liver support therapy was started when the total plasma bilirubin level > 20 mg/dl, or an increase in bilirubin level of more than 2 mg/dl per day for 4 days. When total bilirubin removal is assessed in these therapies, a 25% decrease is considered the optimal value. A greater decrease in bilirubin was seen with PE (35 ± 13%) followed by PAP (30 ± 12%) and the lowest percentage with MARS (24 ± 14%), and the values of transaminases and coagulation tests were not different between the three techniques. In this review, the costs per treatment are mentioned, being the most economical PE, followed by PAP and the most expensive MARS due to equipment and the long time the therapy takes. It is important to mention that an advantage of MARS over the other techniques mentioned is its application in acute kidney injury (AKI) that requires renal support therapy.

11. Double plasma molecular adsorption system

The double plasma molecular adsorption system (DPMAS) modality has the particularity of using a CRRT or intermittent hemodialysis machine with second roller pumps. Once the blood is drawn through the catheter with a blood pump flow of 150 ml/min, the blood passes through a high permeability filter to separate the plasma and then, the separated plasma is driven by a second roller pump at 25–50 ml/min, which enters a first BS330-JAFRON styrene-divinylbenzene cartridge with anion-exchange resin and later the plasma goes through a second HA330 II-JAFRON cartridge with neutral macroporous resin, to then be reconstituted by the plasma in the blood that returns to the patient's catheter (**Figure 10**).

The evidence consulted reports an RCT from China [50], which includes patients with ALF and ACLF. They are randomized into two groups, 20 patients in the SMT and PE group vs. 27 in the SMT and DPMAS group. The result in the primary outcome shows a survival at 4–12 months is similar in both groups (p = 0.887), in the secondary outcomes measurements of bilirubin and CRP are performed, which decrease more

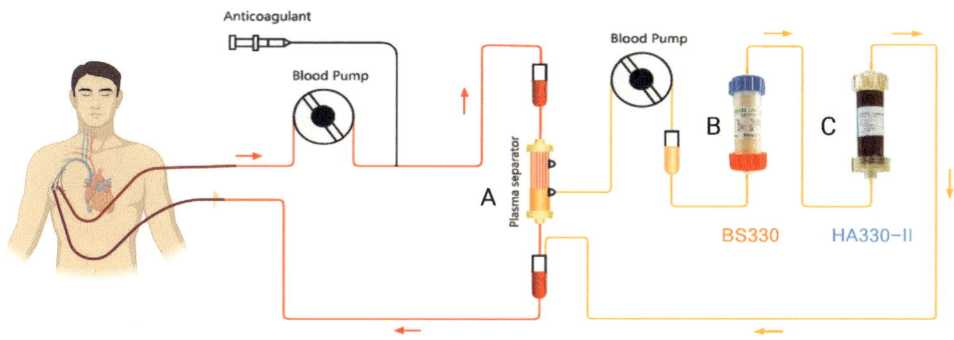

Figure 10.
Double plasma molecular adsorption system (DPMAS). A) The blood extracted through the catheter enters a high permeability filter to separate the plasma. B) The separated plasma is driven by a second roller pump that drives the plasma into a first BS330-JAFRON cartridge made of styrene-divinylbenzene with anion-exchange resin. C) Subsequently, the plasma passes through a second cartridge HA330 II-JAFRON with neutral macroporous resin.

significantly with PE ($p = 0.002$), and the decrease in procalcitonin was similar in both groups, greater hypoalbuminemia in the PE group. The increase in IL-6 is strikingly evident in both groups and is attributed to being a stimulatory factor in liver regeneration.

During a meta-analysis [51] of 11 articles on ACLF due to hepatitis B, where the values of total bilirubin and albumin did not differ in both groups, ALT decreased more in DPMAS+PE than, with PE alone, the levels of I international standardized ratio (INR) and blood platelet (PT) were prolonged, but there were no significant differences between the two groups. In this study, there was a lot of heretogenicity in study quality which could lead to bias.

In another meta-analysis [52] of 11 RCT studies, including 1087 hepatitis B patients with ACLF, comparing two treatment groups with DPMAS + plasma exchange vs. plasma exchange alone, 90-day survival was higher with DPMAS + plasma exchange ($P = < 0.00001$), and bilirubin and alanine aminotransferase values after treatment were lower with DPMAS + PE ($P = < 0.00001$) and ($P = 0.02$), respectively. There was no statistical significance in prothrombin activity (PTA), PT, platelets (PLT), INR, and hemoglobin (HB).

In a retrospective controlled study [53] with DPMAS where 131 with ACLF for hepatitis B were recruited, they were assigned to the plasma exchange group vs. DPMAS + plasma exchange. Low-volume exchange plasma (2–2.4 L) was performed with fresh-frozen plasma in the DPMAS group first and then with exchange plasma. In the DPMAS + plasma exchange group, bilirubin decreases after the procedure, at 24 and 72 hours ($P = < 0.05$), and survival at 28 days was better ($P = 0.043$). Prospective studies are needed to assess long-term survival.

12. Coupled plasma filtration with adsorption

Coupled plasma filtration with adsorption (CPFA) is a technique, which requires a CRRT machine (Amplya), especially designed to combine the separation of plasma from blood by a high-permeability polyethersulfone filter. Then, the separated plasma circulates through a styrene cartridge-divinylbenzene copolymer and the purified plasma is reconstituted with the blood, which is finally returned to a CRRT polyphenylene hemofilter to remove water-soluble molecules (**Figure 11**).

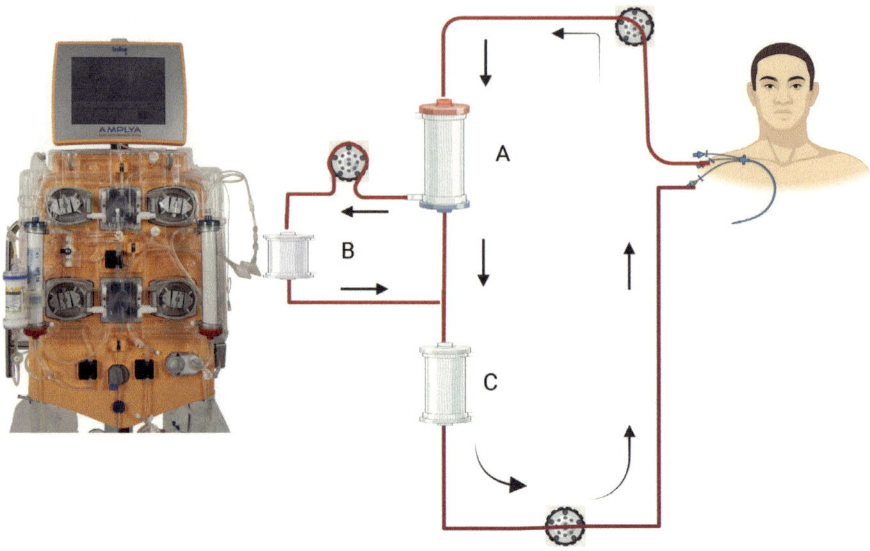

Figure 11.
Coupled plasma filtration with adsorption (CPFA). A) Requires the separation of plasma from blood by a high-permeability polyethersulfone filter. B) The separated plasma is circulated through a styrene-divinylbenzene copolymer cartrige. C) The purified plasma is reconstituted with the blood, which is finally returned to a CRRT polyphenylene hemofilter.

The Hercole trail [54], a non-randomized observational study that included 12 patients, 4 with ALF and 8 with ACLF, started APFC with total bilirubin values > 20 mg/dl and MELD >20 that did not improve with SMT. It is observed that CPFA did not modify the SOFA and MELD score, the decrease in bilirubin ($p = 0.0006$) and bile acids ($p = 0.047$) decreased significantly, but after the third hour, the filter was saturated. Water-soluble molecules, such as water-soluble toxins, urea, and creatinine, did not change significantly before or after PAFC, attributed to low convective volumes, INR and aPTT values were prolonged, but bleeding was not reported. It is important to mention that bilirubin rebound is expected to occur after the first session and ranges from 10 to 40% and is characteristic of the multicompartmental model of bilirubin kinetics, which occurs in any of the aforementioned therapies. It is a promising therapy, which requires further evidence with randomized controlled trials.

13. Hemoperfusion

There are many reports of the use of hemoperfusion in liver failure since the 70s and 80s.

Hemoperfusion is an extracorporeal therapy technique, which allows the passage of blood through a filter with the adsorption capacity of molecules with molecular weights from 5 to 50 kD, and the cartridges are classified according to a) composition in natural compounds (carbons) and synthetics (divinylbenzene), b) surface and volume, c) size, and d) selectivity.

The adsorption mechanisms attract solutes through different forces (hydrophobic interactions, ionic attraction, hydrogen bonding, and Van der Waals interactions), which allow the uptake of PAPMs, DAMPs, cytokines, chemokines, and multiple toxic substances (drugs, poisons).

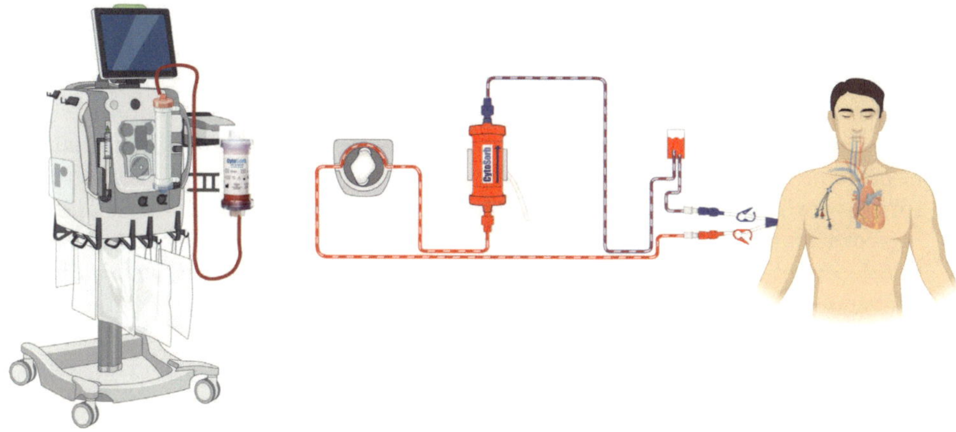

Figure 12.
Hemoperfusion. It is an adsorptive therapy that uses activated carbon cartridges or divinylbenzene resins.

The cartridges can be mounted in CRRT or in an intermittent hemodialysis (IH) machine, and it can be coupled to CRRT, prolonged intermittent renal replacement therapy (PIRRT), or IH modalities, to simultaneously perform both therapies (**Figure 12**).

In a retrospective study [55], the use of charcoal hemoperfusion in 13 patients with refractory pruritus in cholestatic, managed to reduce pruritus in 69% of patients and in a numerical pruritus score performed before the start of therapy with a score of 9/10, decreased to 4/10, with an average of 5 sessions.

Stanje J et al. [56], in an *in vitro* two-compartment model established for the comparison of MARS vs. Cytosorb, water-soluble toxicants, such as creatinine, decreased significantly with MARS ($p = < 0.04$), and the decrease in ammonia was more significant with Cytosorb ($p = < 0.05$). Regarding the toxins bound to albumin, Cytosorb managed to decrease the values of total and indirect bilirubin in statistically significant values ($p = < 0.03$) and the elimination of bile acids was comparable. The decrease in cytokines, such as IL-6 and TNF-α with 6 hours of therapy, was significant with Cytosorb. More controlled studies are required to support the results reported in experimental studies and case series.

14. Hepatorenal syndrome

Patients with advanced cirrhosis frequently show some degree of renal dysfunction, and there is a strong relationship between the severity of cirrhosis and renal dysfunction. It has been estimated that more than 20% of patients hospitalized for acute decompensation of cirrhosis develop acute kidney injury. Cirrhotic patients can develop any type of renal failure, that is, prerenal (41.7%), intrarenal (38%), and postrenal (0.3%) types [57, 58].

Hepatorenal syndrome (HRS) is a peculiar type of functional AKI described in advanced liver disease with ascites and is characterized by vasoconstriction that does not improve with volume replacement. Hepatorenal syndrome accounts for 20% of AKI in patients with cirrhosis. The incidence of HRS in the natural history of cirrhosis is 18% after 1 year and 39% after 5 years [59].

AKI in the cirrhosis spectrum is defined using the KDIGO criteria, and the international ascites club introduces this definition of serum creatinine increase of ≥0.3 mg/dL within 48 hours in hospitalized patients or an increase of ≥50% in 7 days [60].

The multiple mechanisms that condition this pathology, and the following mechanisms are mentioned:

- **Intrahepatic hemodynamics:** Alterations in hepatic architecture conditioned by regeneration, fibrosis, and thrombosis nodules, together with functional alterations due to an imbalance between the greater production of vasoconstrictors (endothelin, leukotriene B4, thromboxane A2, and Angiotensin II) and less formation of local vasodilators (nitric oxide, cannabinoids) determine the development of portal hypertension and splanchnic vasodilation, which allows the sequestration of blood in this territory [61].

- **Hepatorenal reflex:** The presence of sensors in intrahepatic sinusoids that are stimulated based on changes in portal pressure and flow is mentioned. The increase in pressure would condition the sending of a signal by the afferent sympathetic nerve in the direction of the brain and the efferent sympathetic response at the renal level. It causes vasoconstriction of the efferent arteriole [62].

- **Systemic hemodynamics:** It is mentioned that a determining factor is the increase in systemic vasodilators, such as nitric oxide, among others, and the sequestration of blood in the splanchnic territory generates an effective decrease in blood volume that stimulates an increase in cardiac output, in order to restore effective arterial blood volume. When the liver disease progresses, severe portal hypertension develops and, together with bacterial translocation that mediates the release of PAMPs into the circulation, increases the inflammatory response that facilitates greater splanchnic vasodilation, causing a lower effective arterial blood volume and the consequent activation of the renin-angiotensin-aldosterone system, which facilitates the reabsorption of sodium and water, likewise this neurohumoral mechanism favors renal vasoconstriction. It is important to mention that relative hypotension stimulates the non-osmotic release of ADH, favoring the reabsorption of water in the collecting ducts [63].

- **Cirrhotic cardiomyopathy:** It is described in an experimental model [64] that in cirrhotic rats a severe blockage of the contractile capacity is generated by the α-adrenergic agonist isoproterenol and the limited capacity to generate the cAMP that stimulates the second messenger. The β-adrenergic receptor is the main determinant of ventricular contractility and experimental studies show a lower density and function of these receptors in patients with cirrhosis. It has been shown that NO inhibits β-adrenergic receptors, altering cardiac stimulation and decreasing cardiac contractility [65]. Endocannabinoids are also increased in patients with cirrhosis, and they can exert a negative inotropic effect in humans. It is described that the cardiac index <1.5 L and MAP <80 mmHg ($p = < 0.05$) are the predictors of hepatorenal syndrome in a 12-month follow-up [66].

- **Inflammatory response:** In cirrhosis, damaged hepatocytes release DAMPs such as high-mobility group box-1 (HMGB1), histones, and activate Kuppfer cells, leading to the production of proinflammatory mediators such as TNF-α, IL-1α, and IL. -6. These proinflammatory signals are detected by the intestinal immune system, and DAMPs bind to TLRs, intestinal Paneth cells, and dendritic cells. The inflammatory response is not limited to the liver; proinflammatory cytokines leak out and bind to TLR 2–4 in tubular cells, generating a damaging effect at the tubular level [67].

- **Relative adrenal insufficiency:** It is attributed by hormonal depletion in the hypothalamic-pituitary axis, adrenal, inflammatory, or ischemic damage, which is present in 80% of patients with cirrhosis with HRS compared to 30% with normal renal function, and this suggests a hormonal role in the HRS development [62].

- **Intra-abdominal pressure–intra-abdominal hypertension:** An experimental study in mice shows that intra-abdominal pressure from 10 to 20 mmHg is associated with higher levels of urea nitrogen and creatinine and the histological findings found report of tubular obstruction due to casts and inflammation and interstitial edema [62].

See **Figure 13**.

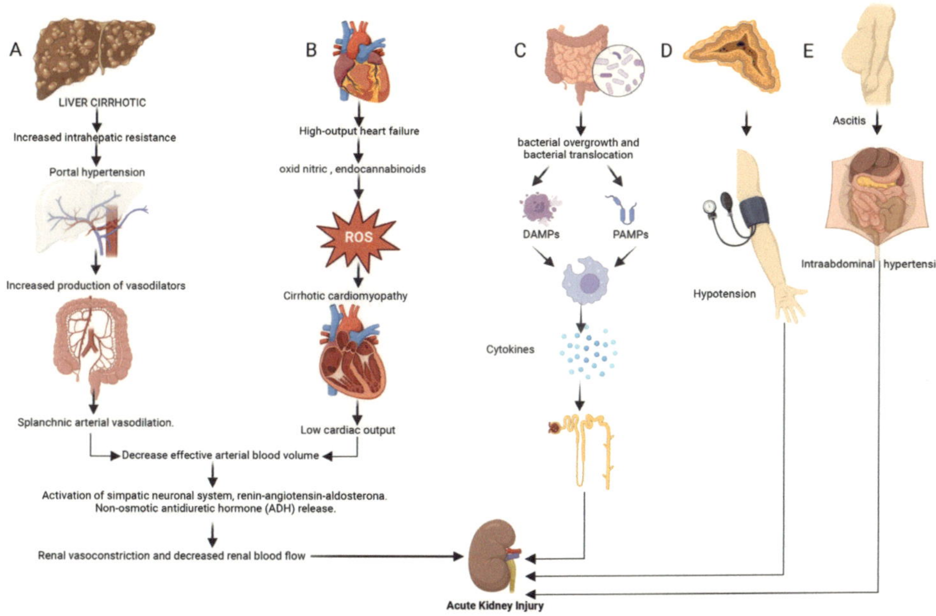

Figure 13.
Pathophysiological mechanisms of hepatorenal syndrome. A) The greater production of vasoconstrictors and less formation of local vasodilators determine the development of portal hypertension and splanchnic vasodilation, which allows the sequestration of blood in this territory. Splanchnic vasodilation generates an effective decrease in blood volume that stimulates an increase in cardiac output, in order to restore effective arterial blood volume. When the liver disease progresses, severe portal hypertension develops and, together with the bacterial translocation that mediates the release of PAMPs into the circulation, increases the inflammatory response that facilitates greater splanchnic vasodilation, causing a lower effective arterial blood volume and the consequent activation of the sympathetic and renin-angiotensin-aldosterone system, which facilitates the reabsorption of sodium and water, B) cirrhotic cardiomyopathy, there are multiple mechanisms that allow its development and condition a decrease in cardiac output, which conditions a decrease in mean arterial pressure, being a predictor of the development of hepatorenal syndrome. C) Bacterial overgrowth and bacterial translocation allow PMAPs to reach the enterohepatic circulation and precipitating factors and the progression of liver damage from the underlying disease allows the release of DAMPS, and both molecular patterns are presented to both Kupffer cells generating an intrahepatic inflammatory response and the presentation of these molecular patterns to dendritic cells and macrophages facilitates SIRS, the arrival of PAMPs and DAMPs to the kidneys allows them to filter and be captured by TLR2-4 of tubular cells, generating a damaging effect. D) Relative adrenal insufficiency that determines hemodynamic changes. E) Increased intra-abdominal pressure due to ascites, associated with changes in intrarenal hemodynamics such as renal venous congestion.

14.1 Diagnosis

The diagnosis of hepatorenal syndrome is difficult and is made by ruling out since there is no laboratory or imaging study to confirm it with certainty.

Within the International Ascites Club criteria, defines AKI as increases in serum creatinine of ≥ 0.3 mg/dL within 48 hours or 50% increase within 7 days in hospitalized patients with no response after 2 days consecutive with the use of albumin (1 g/kg of body weight), in the absence of shock, without the use of nephrotoxic drugs, absence of proteinuria (> 500 mg/day), absence of microhematuria (> 50 red blood cells per high-power field), and normal findings on renal ultrasound [60].

The aforementioned criteria should be reviewed because many patients with cirrhosis usually present hypotension without being in septic shock, and the presence of hematuria and proteinuria may be present secondary to IgA nephropathy or membranoproliferative glomerulonephritis due to C virus, and it should be considered that they are also exposed to use of antibiotics and analgesics. I believe that many of them have overlapping causes within the spectrum of hepatorenal syndrome [68].

In the analysis, there is no pathognomonic marker. In the past, it was reported that FENA <1% was an indicator of this disease; currently, the cutoff value seems to be lower <0.2% [69], in the advent of biomarkers the urinary NGAL <400 μg/L correlates with hepatorenal syndrome, and urinary NAGAL values >400 μg/L occur in acute tubular necrosis (ATN) [70].

14.2 Treatment

The initial treatment of AKI in the spectrum of cirrhosis is the use of albumin (1 g/kg of body weight) for 48 hours. Velez et. al [71] describe AKI phenotypes in cirrhosis based on the diameter of the inferior vena cava (IVC) evaluated by ultrasound, in the aforementioned work three groups are described: group with IVC diameter <1.3 cm, which is subdivided According to CVI collapse, it can be > 40%, which corresponds to the fluid depleted phenotype and this group would benefit from albumin replacement; in those with <40% collapse, it corresponds to the intra-abdominal hypertension phenotype and would benefit from paracentesis. In the second group with IVC 1.3-2 cm corresponds to the fluid repleted phenotype, which would benefit from vasoconstrictors and in the third group corresponds to those with IVC > 2 cm and which is subdivided based on collapse >40% indicating a state of euvolemia, the use of vasoconstrictors would be a good therapeutic option and those with collapsibility <40% correspond to the fluid expanded phenotype where diuretics are indicated.

If after expansion with albumin the decrease in creatinine is not achieved, albumin should be maintained at 20–40 g and add Terlipressin 0.5–1 mg/4–6 hours, titrating the dose with 2-mg increment every day until reaching a maximum dose of 12 mg, an adequate response is defined when a 25% drop in initial creatinine is achieved, and in case of no response, Terlipressin can be administered for 14 days. It is recommended that infusion is better when compared with boluses every 6 hours. The predictive factors of poor response to Terlipressin are elevated total bilirubin values >10 mg/dl, lack of MAP increase of 5 mmHg on day 3, as well as NGAL >728 μg/L. (61.63).

The evidence on Terlipressin, norepinephrine, octreotide, and midodrine is extensive and exceeds the scope of the review.

15. Renal support therapies in hepatorenal syndrome

The use of renal supportive therapy is indicated when patients with hepatorenal syndrome develop absolute indications for renal supportive therapy (RST) (severe metabolic acidosis, severe hyperkalemia, fluid overload, encephalopathy, and uremia) in nonresponders to the use of Terlipressin with albumin.

AKI, due to HRS and ATN, has a poor prognosis because 40% require RST and 60% die within 90 days [72]. In a retrospective cohort of 472 patients with diagnoses of HRS and ATN, 341 of these did not enter the waiting list and 131 were included on the waiting list. It was evident that those who developed HRS presented higher SOFA and MELD scores and patients with ATN presented sepsis and required vasopressors and mechanical ventilation. The 6-month survival for those who were not placed on the waiting list with HRS (84%) and ATN (85%) was similar. The RST start is controversial in patients who are not candidates for liver transplantation because it does not modify the prognosis.

At this point, three scenarios are proposed [73]:

1. The patient is included in the waiting list and the need for RST becomes a bridge until the transplant, in this case, there is no doubt of the benefit.

2. The second scenario is a patient in the evaluation phase for liver transplantation, where the need for RST will be until the inclusion on the list is clear.

3. In those who are not included on the waiting list for liver transplantation, can receive RST temporarily or until the experts in palliative care, the patient and the family decide they will limit efforts in a terminal illness.

16. Conclusions

ALF and ACLF represent very complex pathophysiological diseases that encompass multiple inflammation mechanisms that perpetuate liver damage and medical treatment is not successful in limiting the damage. The use of albumin-based extracorporeal support therapies has not been shown to have an impact on survival and we see plasma exchange therapies or therapies combined with hemoperfusion show better survival than the traditional ones, although more randomized controlled trials with a greater number of patients are needed of patients to have a stronger recommendation.

Hepatorenal syndrome is a renal complication in patients with advanced liver cirrhosis and is triggered by multiple mechanisms. There is no gold standard for diagnosis, which is by exclusion, albumin and Terlipressin therapy is the recommended treatment in response to treatment with higher mortality, which is not modified by the use of renal support therapies.

Author details

Maiko Alejandro Tavera Díaz
Nephrology Department, Univalle Hospital, Bolivia

*Address all correspondence to: taveradiaz@gmail.com

References

[1] Asrani SK, Devarbhavi H, Eaton J, Kamath PS, et al. Burden of liver diseases in the world. Journal of Hepatology. 2019;**70**(1):151-171. Available from: DOI: 10.1016/j.jhep.2018.09.014

[2] Sarin SK, Choudhury A, et al. Acute-on-chronic liver failure. Current Gastroenterology Reports. 2016;**18**(12):61. Available from: DOI: 10.1007/s11894-016-0535-8

[3] Weiler N, Schlotmann A, Schnitzbauer AA, Zeuzem S, Welker MW, et al. The epidemiology of acute liver failure. Deutsches Ärzteblatt International. 2020;**117**(4):43-50. Available from: DOI: 10.3238/arztebl.2020.0043

[4] Stravitz RT, Lee WM, et al. Acute liver failure. Lancet. 2019;**394**(10201):869-881. Available from: DOI: 10.1016/s0140-6736(19)31894-x

[5] Bernal W, Wendon J, et al. Acute liver failure. The New England Journal of Medicine. 2013;**369**(26):2525-2534. Available from: DOI: 10.1056/NEJMra1208937

[6] Arroyo V, Moreau R, Kamath PS, Jalan R, Ginès P, Nevens F, et al. Acute-on-chronic liver failure in cirrhosis. Nature Reviews. Disease Primers. 2016;**2**(1):16041. Available from: DOI: 10.1038/nrdp.2016.41

[7] Bernal W, Jalan R, Quaglia A, Simpson K, Wendon J, Burroughs A, et al. Acute-on-chronic liver failure. Lancet. 2015;**386**(10003):1576-1587. Available from: DOI: 10.1016/S0140-6736(15)00309-8

[8] Arroyo V, Moreau R, Jalan R, et al. Acute-on-chronic liver failure. The New England Journal of Medicine. 2020;**382**(22):2137-2145. Available from: DOI: 10.1056/NEJMra1914900

[9] Bernsmeier C, Antoniades CG, Wendon J, et al. What's new in acute liver failure? Intensive Care Medicine. 2014;**40**(10):1545-1548. Available from: DOI: 10.1007/s00134-014-3350-4

[10] Craig DG, Lee P, Pryde EA, Hayes PC, Simpson KJ, et al. Serum neopterin and soluble CD163 as markers of macrophage activation in paracetamol (acetaminophen)-induced human acute liver injury. Alimentary Pharmacology & Therapeutics. 2013;**38**(11-12):1395-1404. DOI: 10.1111/apt.12530

[11] European Association for the Study of the Liver Clinical practice guidelines panel, Wendon J, Panel members, Cordoba J, Dhawan A, et al. EASL clinical practical guidelines on the management of acute (fulminant) liver failure. Journal of Hepatology. 2017;**66**(5):1047-1081. [Internet] Available from: DOI: 10.1016/j.jhep.2016.12.003

[12] Sarin SK, Choudhury A. Acute-on-chronic liver failure: Terminology, mechanisms and management. Nature Reviews. Gastroenterology & Hepatology. 2016;**13**(3):131-149. Available from: DOI: 10.1038/nrgastro.2015.219

[13] Honore PM, Hoste E, Molnár Z, Jacobs R, Joannes-Boyau O, Malbrain MLNG, et al. Cytokine removal in human septic shock: Where are we and where are we going? Annals of Intensive Care. 2019;**9**(1):1-13. Available from: DOI: 10.1186/s13613-019-0530-y

[14] Carvalho JR, Machado MV, et al. New insights about albumin and

liver disease. Annals of Hepatology. 2018;**17**(4):547-560. Available from: DOI: 10.5604/01.3001.0012.0916

[15] Oettl K, Marsche G, et al. Redox state of human serum albumin in terms of cysteine-34 in health and disease. Methods in Enzymology. 2010;**474**:181-195. Available from: DOI: 10.1016/S0076-6879(10)74011-8

[16] Sun L, Yin H, Liu M, Xu G, Zhou X, Ge P, et al. Impaired albumin function: A novel potential indicator for liver function damage? Annals of Medicine. 2019;**51**(7-8):333-344. Available from: DOI: 10.1080/07853890.2019.1693056.

[17] Bernardi M, Angeli P, Claria J, Moreau R, Gines P, Jalan R, et al. Albumin in decompensated cirrhosis: New concepts and perspectives. Gut. 2020;**69**(6):1127-1138. Available from: DOI: 10.1136/gutjnl-2019-318843

[18] Alcaraz-Quiles J, Casulleras M, Oettl K, Titos E, Flores-Costa R, Duran-Güell M, et al. Oxidized albumin triggers a cytokine storm in leukocytes through P38 mitogen-activated protein kinase: Role in systemic inflammation in decompensated cirrhosis. Hepatology. 2018;**68**(5):1937-1952 Available from: https://pubmed.ncbi.nlm.nih.gov/30070728/

[19] Oettl K, Stadlbauer V, Krisper P, Stauber RE, et al. Effect of extracorporeal liver support by molecular adsorbents recirculating system and Prometheus on redox state of albumin in acute-on-chronic liver failure. Therapeutic Apheresis and Dialysis: Official Peer-Reviewed Journal of the International Society for Apheresis, the Japanese Society for Apheresis, the Japanese Society for Dialysis Therapy. 2009;**13**(5):431-436. Available from: DOI: 10.1111/j.1744-9987.2009.00762.x

[20] Jalan R, Schnurr K, Mookerjee RP, Sen S, Cheshire L, Hodges S, et al. Alterations in the functional capacity of albumin in patients with decompensated cirrhosis is associated with increased mortality. Hepatology. 2009;**50**(2):555-564. Available from: DOI: 10.1002/hep.22913

[21] Groeneveld D, Cline-Fedewa H, Baker KS, Williams KJ, Roth RA, Mittermeier K, et al. Von Willebrand factor delays liver repair after acetaminophen-induced acute liver injury in mice. Journal of Hepatology. 2020;**72**(1):146-155. Available from: DOI: 10.1016/j.jhep.2019.09.030

[22] Hugenholtz GCG, Adelmeijer J, Meijers JCM, Porte RJ, Stravitz RT, Lisman T, et al. An imbalance between von Willebrand factor and ADAMTS13 in acute liver failure. Hepatology. 2013;**58**(2):752-761. Available from: DOI: 10.1002/hep.26372

[23] Gustafson E, Hamad OA, Deckmyn H, Barbu A, Ekdahl KN, Nilsson B, et al. Exposure of von Willebrand factor on isolated hepatocytes promotes tethering of platelets to the cell surface. Transplantation. 2019;**103**(8):1630-1638. Available from: DOI: 10.1097/TP.0000000000002707

[24] Prasanna KS, Goel A, Amirtharaj GJ, Ramachandran A, Balasubramanian KA, Mackie I, et al. Plasma von Willebrand factor levels predict in-hospital survival in patients with acute-on-chronic liver failure. Indian Journal of Gastroenterology. 2016;**35**(6):432-440. Available from: DOI: 10.1007/s12664-016-0708-2-

[25] Groeneveld DJ, Poole LG, Luyendyk JP, et al. Targeting von Willebrand factor in liver diseases: A novel therapeutic strategy? Journal of Thrombosis and Haemostasis. 2021;**19**(6):1390-1408. Available from: DOI: 10.1111/jth.15312

[26] Roth K, Strickland J, Copple BL, et al. Regulation of macrophage activation in the liver after acute injury: Role of the fibrinolytic system. World Journal of Gastroenterology. 2020;**26**(16):1879-1887. Available from: DOI: 10.3748/wjg.v26.i16.1879

[27] Nielsen MC, Hvidbjerg Gantzel R, Clària J, Trebicka J, Møller HJ, Grønbæk H, et al. Macrophage activation markers, CD163 and CD206, in acute-on-chronic liver failure. Cell. 2020;**9**(5):1175. Available from: DOI: 10.3390/cells9051175

[28] Chamuleau RA. Future of bioartificial liver support. World Journal of Gastrointestinal Surgery. 2009;**1**(1):21-25. Available from: DOI: 10.4240/wjgs.v1.i1.21

[29] Mitzner SR, Stange J, Klamt S, Koball S, Hickstein H, Reisinger EC. Albumin dialysis MARS: Knowledge from 10 years of clinical investigation. ASAIO Journal 2009 2022; 55(5):498-502. Available from: https://pubmed.ncbi.nlm.nih.gov/19730006/.

[30] Tandon R, Froghi S, et al. Artificial liver support systems. Journal of Gastroenterology and Hepatology. 2021;**36**(5):1164-1179. Available from: DOI: 10.1111/jgh.15255

[31] Saliba F, Camus C, Durand F, Mathurin P, Letierce A, Delafosse B, et al. Albumin dialysis with a noncell artificial liver support device in patients with acute liver failure: A randomized, controlled trial: A randomized, controlled trial. Annals of Internal Medicine. 2013;**159**(8):522-531. Available from: DOI: 10.7326/0003-4819-159-8-201310150-00005

[32] Bañares R, Nevens F, Larsen FS, Jalan R, Albillos A, Dollinger M, et al. Extracorporeal albumin dialysis with the molecular adsorbent recirculating system in acute-on-chronic liver failure: The RELIEF trial. Hepatology. 2013;**57**(3):1153-1162. Available from: DOI: 10.1002/hep.26185

[33] Vaid A, Chweich H, Balk EM, Jaber BL. Molecular adsorbent recirculating system as artificial support therapy for liver failure: A meta-analysis: A meta-analysis. ASAIO Journal (American Society for Artificial Internal Organs: 2012). 2012;**58**(1):51-59. Available from. DOI: 10.1097/MAT.0b013e31823fd077

[34] Bañares R, Ibáñez-Samaniego L, Torner JM, Pavesi M, Olmedo C, Catalina MV, et al. Meta-analysis of individual patient data of albumin dialysis in acute-on-chronic liver failure: Focus on treatment intensity. Therapeutic Advances in Gastroenterology. 2019;**12**:1756284819879565. Available from: DOI: 10.1177/1756284819879565

[35] Saliba F, Bañares R, Larsen FS, Wilmer A, Parés A, Mitzner S, et al. Artificial liver support in patients with liver failure: A modified DELPHI consensus of international experts. Intensive Care Medicine. 2022;**48**(10):1352-1367. Available from: DOI: 10.1007/s00134-022-06802-1

[36] Kribben A, Gerken G, Haag S, Herget-Rosenthal S, Treichel U, Betz C, et al. Effects of fractionated plasma separation and adsorption on survival in patients with acute-on-chronic liver failure. Gastroenterology. 2012;**142**(4):782-789.e3. Available from: DOI: 10.1053/j.gastro.2011.12.056

[37] Stadlbauer V, Krisper P, Aigner R, Haditsch B, Jung A, Lackner C, et al. Effect of extracorporeal liver support by MARS and Prometheus on serum cytokines in acute-on-chronic liver failure. Critical Care. 2006;**10**(6):R169. Available from: DOI: 10.1186/cc5119

[38] Sen S, Davies NA, Mookerjee RP, Cheshire LM, Hodges SJ, Williams R, et al. Pathophysiological effects of albumin dialysis in acute-on-chronic liver failure: A randomized controlled study.

Liver Transplantation, Available from. 2004;**10**:1109-1119. DOI: 10.1002/lt.20236

[39] Rifai K, Ernst T, Kretschmer U, Haller H, Manns MP, Fliser D. Removal selectivity of Prometheus: A new extracorporeal liver support device. World Journal of Gastroenterology. 2006;**12**:940-944. Available from: DOI: 10.3748/wjg.v12.i6.940

[40] Sponholz C, Matthes K, Rupp D, Backaus W, Klammt S, Karailieva D, et al. Molecular adsorbent recirculating system and single-pass albumin dialysis in liver failure--a prospective, randomized crossover study. Critical Care. 2016;**20**(1):2. Available from: DOI: 10.1186/s13054-015-1159-3

[41] Benyoub K, Muller M, Bonnet A, Simon R, Gazon M, Duperret S, et al. Amounts of bile acids and bilirubin removed during single-pass albumin dialysis in patients with liver failure: Letters to the editor. Therapeutic Apheresis and Dialysis. 2011;**15**(5): 504-506. Available from: https://pubmed.ncbi.nlm.nih.gov/21974706/

[42] Wallon G, Guth C, Guichon C, Thevenon S, Gazon M, Viale J-P, et al. Extracorporeal albumin dialysis in liver failure with MARS and SPAD: A randomized crossover trial. Blood Purification. 2022;**51**(3):243-250. Available from: DOI: 10.1159/000515825

[43] Stahl K, Schmidt JJ, Seeliger B, Schmidt BMW, Welte T, Haller H, et al. Effect of therapeutic plasma exchange on endothelial activation and coagulation-related parameters in septic shock. Critical Care. 2020, 2020;**24**(1):71. Available from. DOI: 10.1186/s13054-020-2799-5

[44] Larsen FS, Schmidt LE, Bernsmeier C, Rasmussen A, Isoniemi H, Patel VC, et al. High-volume plasma exchange in patients with acute liver failure: An open randomized controlled trial. Journal of Hepatology. 2016;**64**(1):69-78. Available from: DOI: 10.1016/j.jhep.2015.08.018

[45] Maiwall R, Bajpai M, Singh A, Agarwal T, Kumar G, Bharadwaj A, et al. Standard-volume plasma exchange improves outcomes in patients with acute liver failure: A randomized controlled trial. Clinical Gastroenterology and Hepatology: The Official Clinical Practice Journal of the American Gastroenterological Association. 2022;**20**(4):e831-e854. Available from: DOI: 10.1016/j.cgh.2021.01.036

[46] Kumar SE, Goel A, Zachariah U, Nair SC, David VG, Varughese S, et al. Low volume plasma exchange and low dose steroid improve survival in patients with alcohol-related acute on chronic liver failure and severe alcoholic hepatitis - preliminary experience. Journal of Clinical and Experimental Hepatology. 2022;**12**(2):372-378. Available from: DOI: 10.1016/j.jceh.2021.07.010

[47] Ocskay K, Kanjo A, Gede N, Szakács Z, Pár G, Erőss B, et al. Uncertainty in the impact of liver support systems in acute-on-chronic liver failure: A systematic review and network meta-analysis. Annals of Intensive Care. 2021;**11**(1):10 Available from: https://pubmed.ncbi.nlm.nih.gov/33462764/

[48] Du L, Ma Y, Zhou S, Chen F, Xu Y, Wang M, et al. A prognostic score for patients with acute-on-chronic liver failure treated with plasma exchange-centered artificial liver support system. Scientific Reports. 2021;**11**(1):1469 Available from: https://www.nature.com/articles/s41598-021-81019-8

[49] Viggiano D, de Pascale E, Marinelli G, Pluvio C, et al. A comparison among three different apheretic techniques for treatment of hyperbilirubinemia. Journal of artificial

organs: The official journal of the Japanese society for. Artificial Organs. 2018;**21**(1):110-116. Available from: DOI: 10.1007/s10047-017-0986-1

[50] Wan Y-M, Li Y-H, Xu Z-Y, Yang J, Yang L-H, Xu Y, et al. Therapeutic plasma exchange versus double plasma molecular absorption system in hepatitis B virus-infected acute-on-chronic liver failure treated by entercavir: A prospective study. Journal of Clinical Apheresis. 2017;**32**(6):453-461. Available from: DOI: 10.1002/jca.21535

[51] Ma L, Zhang X, Ma W, Ding X, et al. Meta-analysis of the efficacy of DPMAS-based artificial liver in the treatment of ACLF. Research Square. 28 April 2022. Available from: https://doi.org/10.21203/rs.3.rs-1604197/v1

[52] Bai W, Yao C, Mao D, Wu J, Wang K, Wei H, et al. The clinical efficacy of double plasma molecular absorption system combined with plasma exchange in the treatment of acute-on-chronic liver failure: A systematic review and meta-analysis. Journal of Healthcare Engineering. 2022;**2022**:3139929 Available from: https://pubmed.ncbi.nlm.nih.gov/35368957/

[53] Yao J, Li S, Zhou L, Luo L, Yuan L, Duan Z, et al. Therapeutic effect of double plasma molecular adsorption system and sequential half-dose plasma exchange in patients with HBV-related acute-on-chronic liver failure. Journal of Clinical Apheresis. 2019;**34**(4):392-398 Available from: https://pubmed.ncbi.nlm.nih.gov/30758886/

[54] Donati G, Angeletti A, Gasperoni L, Piscaglia F, Croci Chiocchini AL, Scrivo A, et al. Detoxification of bilirubin and bile acids with intermittent coupled plasmafiltration and adsorption in liver failure (HERCOLE study). Journal of Nephrology. 2021;**34**(1):77-88. Available from: DOI: 10.1007/s40620-020-00799-w

[55] Ronco C, Bellomo R. Sorbents: From Basic Structure to Clinical Application. In: Ronco C, Bellomo R, editors. Critical Care Nephrology. Elsevier Health Sciences. 2017:1137-1154.e2

[56] Kittanamongkolchai W, El-Zoghby ZM, Eileen Hay J, Wiesner RH, Kamath PS, LaRusso NF, et al. Charcoal hemoperfusion in the treatment of medically refractory pruritus in cholestatic liver disease. Hepatology International. 2017;**11**(4):384-389. Available from: DOI: 10.1007/s12072-016-9775-9

[57] Dominik A, Stange J, et al. Similarities, differences, and potential synergies in the mechanism of action of albumin dialysis using the MARS albumin dialysis device and the CytoSorb hemoperfusion device in the treatment of liver failure. Blood Purification. 2021;**50**(1):119-128. Available from: DOI: 10.1159/000508810

[58] Angeli P, Merkel C, et al. Pathogenesis and management of hepatorenal syndrome in patients with cirrhosis. Journal of Hepatology. 2008;**48**(Suppl. 1):S93-S103. Available from: DOI: 10.1016/j.jhep.2008.01.010

[59] Ginès A, Escorsell A, Ginès P, Saló J, Jiménez W, Inglada L, et al. Incidence, predictive factors, and prognosis of the hepatorenal syndrome in cirrhosis with ascites. Gastroenterology. 1993;**105**(1):229-236. Available from: DOI: 10.1016/0016-5085(93)90031-7

[60] Angeli P, Garcia-Tsao G, Nadim MK, Parikh CR, et al. News in pathophysiology, definition and classification of hepatorenal syndrome: A step beyond the International Club of Ascites (ICA) consensus document. Journal of Hepatology. 2019;**71**(4):811-822. Available from: DOI: 10.1016/j.jhep.2019.07.002

[61] Martell M, Coll M, Ezkurdia N, Raurell I, Genescà J, et al. Physiopathology

of splanchnic vasodilation in portal hypertension. World. Journal of Hepatology. 2010;**2**(6):208-220. Available from: DOI: 10.4254/wjh.v2.i6.208

[62] Hasan I, Rashid T, Chirila RM, Ghali P, Wadei HM, et al. Hepatorenal syndrome: Pathophysiology and evidence-based management update. Revue Roumaine de. Médecine Interne. 2021;**59**(3):227-261. Available from: DOI: 10.2478/rjim-2021-0006

[63] Ginès P, Schrier RW, et al. Renal failure in cirrhosis. The New England Journal of Medicine. 2009;**361**(13):1279-1290. Available from: DOI: 10.1056/NEJMra0809139

[64] Ward CA, Liu H, Lee SS, et al. Altered cellular calcium regulatory systems in a rat model of cirrhotic cardiomyopathy. Gastroenterology. 2001;**121**(5):1209-1218. Available from: DOI: 10.1053/gast.2001.28653

[65] Bernardi M. Cirrhotic cardiomyopathy. Clinics in Liver Disease. 2013;**2**(3):99-101. Available from: DOI: 10.1002/cld.141

[66] Krag A, Bendtsen F, Henriksen JH, Møller S, et al. Low cardiac output predicts development of hepatorenal syndrome and survival in patients with cirrhosis and ascites. Gut. 2010;**59**(1):105-110. Available from: DOI: 10.1136/gut.2009.180570

[67] Fukazawa K, Lee HT, et al. Updates on hepato-renal syndrome. Journal of Anesthesia & Clinical Research. 2013;**4**(9):352. Available from: DOI: 10.4172/2155-6148.1000352

[68] Velez JCQ, Therapondos G, Juncos LA, et al. Reappraising the spectrum of AKI and hepatorenal syndrome in patients with cirrhosis. Nature reviews. Nephrology. 2020;**16**(3):137-155. Available from: DOI: 10.1038/s41581-019-0218-4

[69] Varghese V, Rivera MS, Alalwan A, Alghamdi AM, Ramanand A, Khan SM, et al. Concomitant identification of muddy brown granular casts and low fractional excretion of urinary sodium in AKI. Kidney 360. 2022;**3**(4):627-635. Available from: DOI: 10.34067/KID.0005692021

[70] Yang CC, Hsieh SC, Li KJ, Wu CH, Lu MC, Tsai CY, et al. Urinary neutrophil gelatinase-associated lipocalin is a potential biomarker for renal damage in patients with systemic lupus erythematosus. Journal of Biomedicine & Biotechnology. 2012;**2012**:759313 Available from: https://pubmed.ncbi.nlm.nih.gov/22500106

[71] Velez JCQ, Petkovich B, Karakala N, Huggins JT et al. Point-of-care echocardiography reveals misclassification of acute kidney injury as hepatorenal syndrome. American Journal of Nephrology 2019;**50**(3): 204-211. Available from: doi:10.1159/000501299

[72] Allegretti AS, Parada XV, Eneanya ND, Gilligan H, Xu D, Zhao S, et al. Prognosis of patients with cirrhosis and AKI who initiate RRT. Clinical Journal of the American Society of Nephrology. 2018;**13**(1):16-25. Available from: DOI: 10.2215/CJN.03610417

[73] JCQ V. Patients with hepatorenal syndrome should be dialyzed? PRO. Kidney 360. 2021;**2**(3):406-409 Available from: http://kidney360.asnjournals.org/content/2/3/406.abstract